Story Treasures

ALSO BY ARTHUR LAZARUS

Neuroleptic Malignant Syndrome and Related Conditions (co-author)

Controversies in Managed Mental Health Care

Career Pathways in Psychiatry: Transition in Changing Times

MD/MBA: Physicians on the New Frontier of Medical Management

*Every Story Counts: Exploring Contemporary
Practice Through Narrative Medicine*

Medicine on Fire: A Narrative Travelogue

Narrative Medicine: The Fifth Vital Sign

Narrative Medicine: Harnessing the Power of Storytelling through Essays

Story Treasures

Medical Essays and Insights in the Narrative Tradition

ARTHUR LAZARUS, MD, MBA

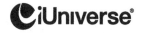

STORY TREASURES
MEDICAL ESSAYS AND INSIGHTS IN THE NARRATIVE TRADITION

iUniverse books may be ordered through booksellers or by contacting:

iUniverse
1663 Liberty Drive
Bloomington, IN 47403
www.iuniverse.com
844-349-9409

ISBN: 978-1-6632-6645-3 (sc)
ISBN: 978-1-6632-6646-0 (e)

Library of Congress Control Number: 2024918111

Print information available on the last page.

iUniverse rev. date: 09/03/2024

To my former patients,
Your stories have been my greatest teachers, and
your courage, my deepest inspiration.

"Medicine...begins with storytelling."

— Siddhartha Mukherjee,
The Emperor of All Maladies: A Biography of Cancer

CONTENTS

SECTION 2: INSIGHTS

AFTERWORD

PREFACE

In the realm of medicine, the pursuit of knowledge is both a scientific endeavor and a deeply human journey. *Story Treasures: Medical Essays and Insights in the Narrative Tradition* is born out of this dual nature, aiming to bridge the gap between clinical and personal experiences that shape healthcare practice.

This book is a compilation of essays and reflections that capture the essence of these experiences. Each story is a pearl, offering a glimpse into the challenges, triumphs, and moments of introspection that define the medical profession and life as a whole. These stories are not merely anecdotes from my career; they are reflections on life, the essence of being, and the universal quest for meaning in times of uncertainty.

Through these pages, I have attempted to share not only the scientific knowledge and clinical insights that have been acquired over years of practice and management but also the emotional and ethical dimensions of medicine. The narratives within are drawn from real-life encounters, testifying to the strength and vulnerability of both patients and healthcare practitioners.

Story Treasures is intended for a diverse readership: healthcare professionals seeking solace and solidarity, patients and families looking for understanding and hope, and anyone curious about the intersections between medicine and the human condition. It is my hope that these essays will inspire, educate, and perhaps even comfort those who read them. The narratives are written with the belief that understanding and empathy are as crucial to medicine as any technological advancement or scientific discovery.

Medicine, at its core, is a deeply human endeavor. It is a field where knowledge and empathy must coexist, where every diagnosis is a story, and every patient history a chapter in a larger narrative. Through these essays and insights, I aim to share not only the intellectual and technical aspects of medical practice but also the emotional and philosophical dimensions that often remain hidden from public view—for example, career turmoil; generational conflict; artificial intelligence; and ethical and leadership challenges, to name a few.

Story Treasures is ultimately a tribute to the healing power of storytelling in medicine. It is an invitation to pause, reflect, and appreciate the intricate dance between health and illness, life and death, joy and sorrow. I hope that readers will find within these pages not only a deeper understanding of the medical world but also a renewed appreciation for the resilience and beauty of the human spirit.

In crafting this collection, I have been guided by a single principle: that every patient has a story worth telling, and every experience holds a lesson worth learning. It is my sincere hope that readers will find these narratives as enriching and enlightening as I have found the experiences that inspired them—ones that compelled me to write each essay as if it were a treasure, and each insight as a gem. As you embark on this journey, may these essays and insights inspire, comfort, and provoke thought. May they collectively remind us all of the preciousness of life and the enduring strength of the human heart.

SECTION 1

Essays

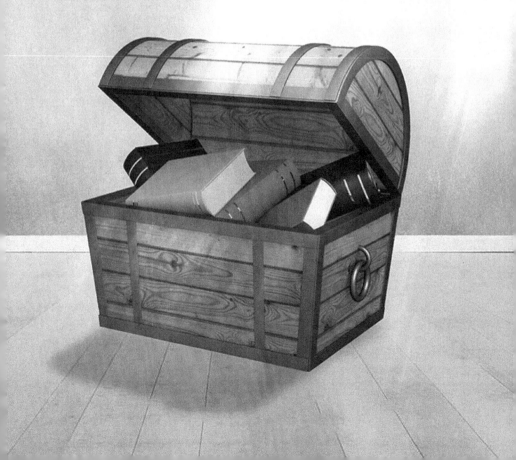

1

The Princess and the Pauper

Both deserve privacy and the sanctity of
space during a course of illness.

The sad news of Princess Kate Middleton's cancer diagnosis is a sound reminder of the sanctity of a person's health status and their right to privacy.

I wasn't sure which adjective I should use to describe Kate's diagnosis—"sad," "tragic," or "devastating." All are equally true, depending on whose perspective you consider. No doubt a cancer diagnosis is "sad" in the public's eyes but even harsher in Kate's. In my opinion, only Kate's viewpoint matters here. Why should the public have a right to know any details of her diagnosis or even that she has cancer?

Kate revealed her health status only as a result of a public frenzy for information. In her now viral video declaration that aired March 22, 2024 she acknowledged what the public had long suspected, that she has been ill since her abdominal surgery in December 2023. However, mounting public pressure forced Kate to unveil her diagnosis. Good for her that she still maintained a semblance of control by not revealing the type of cancer, stating only that she was in the early stages of "preventive chemotherapy."

Between December and March, the royals were hounded by the press, for example, to explain why the notorious photo of Kate and her children had been altered—she preferred to use the term "edited"—and who was behind the attempt to access her medical records while in the hospital. Newsworthy sources tended to blame the general public and 5 billion internet users who basically forced the royals into disclosure and, alternatively, to Kensington Palace for being so coy thinking they could hide the truth.

But whose truth are we talking about? There is only one set of medical facts to explain Kate's condition, and those facts belong to her and no one else. The roots of medical privacy are deep, dating back to the ancient Greeks. The Hippocratic Oath, which doctors still swear by today, includes a pledge to respect the privacy of patients and keep their information confidential.

Despite the early acknowledgment of the importance of privacy in healthcare, it wasn't until the advent of modern technology that the need for formal laws and regulations became apparent. As healthcare systems began to keep electronic records and share information across networks, the potential for breaches in patient privacy increased dramatically.

In the U.S., the Health Insurance Portability and Accountability Act (HIPAA), enacted in 1996, was a landmark piece of legislation designed to address these concerns. HIPAA established national standards for the protection of certain health information and set guidelines for the use and disclosure of patients' health records. It also gave patients the right to access their own medical records and request corrections.

The origin of HIPAA can be traced back to the early 1990s, when healthcare providers started to move away from paper records and adopt electronic health record systems. This transition raised concerns about the security and privacy of patient information. In response, Congress passed HIPAA, with a key provision known as the Privacy Rule.

The Privacy Rule, which went into effect in 2003, set standards for the protection of individuals' medical records and other personal health information. It applies to health plans, healthcare clearinghouses, and those healthcare providers that conduct certain healthcare transactions electronically.

Over time, the concept of medical privacy has evolved from an ethical guideline to a legally enforceable standard, reflecting the ever-changing landscape of healthcare and technology. The only problem is that the law is aimed primarily at those working in the healthcare profession or tangentially to it. It does not deter the public from unscrupulous means to discover the circumstances behind a celebrity's health status, or to quench their insatiable thirst for answers that can only be obtained by invading someone's privacy.

The situation with Kate is reminiscent of the undertakings surrounding the Judd family in 2022. Following the suicide death of country singer Naomi, her daughter and actress Ashley published an essay in the *New York Times* detailing her stance against Tennessee laws that could publicize investigation files about her mother's death. "This profoundly intimate personal and medical information does not belong in the press, on the internet or anywhere except in our memories," she shared.

Subsequently, a bill was proposed in the Tennessee legislature to limit access to death records, photographs, investigative reports, and 9-1-1 calls if law enforcement determines the death was not the result of a crime. However, the bill has yet to see the light of day, receiving pushback from lobbyists, many of them representing the media.

Madelyn Gould, PhD, MPH, the Irving Philips professor of epidemiology (in psychiatry) at Columbia University Medical Center, has extensively documented the phenomenon of suicide contagion for media coverage and was cited by Judd in her attempts to keep the media out of her family's private affairs. Gould's research has found an association of celebrity suicide reporting with increases in suicide, known as the Werther effect.

The "contagion" appears to have spread to other diagnoses, including cancer, and has targeted individuals other than celebrities and royals.

Kate's current misfortune is eerily similar to Princess Diana's death in that it was largely related to the paparazzi. At the time of her death, "Princess Di" was a private citizen. The vehicle that she was traveling in was being pursued by photographers. The ensuing accident caused her death. This incident resulted in stricter laws and guidelines being implemented around the world to protect the privacy and safety of individuals from intrusive media practices.

An official spokesperson said that Kate and William were extremely moved by the global response to her cancer diagnosis while also reiterating their plea for privacy. You can point as many fingers as you want at Kensington Palace, mainstream newspapers, social media and the general public outcry for telling the truth (or concealing it), but the fact is no person—princess or pauper—should have to beg for their health privacy.

2

Lies, Damned Lies, and Statistics.

Common pitfalls underlying cause-and-effect relationships.

In the realm of medicine, cause and effect relationships are those where a specific cause, such as a disease, condition, or treatment, directly leads to a specific outcome or effect. An example of this is the established fact that smoking causes lung cancer. Similarly, it is well-documented that regular, heavy alcohol consumption directly leads to liver cirrhosis.

On the other hand, phrases like "associated with," "linked to" and "tied to" denote a correlation or relationship between two factors, but do not definitively establish causality. For instance, a sedentary lifestyle is often associated with heart disease. This means that a higher incidence of heart disease is observed in people who lead an inactive lifestyle, but it does not necessarily establish that a sedentary lifestyle is the direct cause of heart disease. Other factors may also contribute to the development of this condition.

Similarly, high stress levels are linked to insomnia. Although people with high stress levels often suffer from insomnia, it is not definitively proven that stress is the direct cause of insomnia, as other factors could also be involved. We might also say that high sugar consumption is associated with obesity. While there is a correlation between the two, it cannot be definitively said that high sugar consumption is the sole or primary cause of obesity, as there are many other contributing factors such as physical inactivity, genetics, and other dietary habits.

Therefore, the difference between cause and effect and phrases like "associated with" and "tied to" essentially lies in the strength and certainty of the relationship. Cause and effect indicate a direct and certain relationship, while "associated with" and "linked to" indicate a correlation or consistent relationship, but not necessarily a direct causal one.

Historically, there are several notable examples where cause and effect relationships in medical science were later proven to be incorrect. One such example is the miasma theory, which proposed that diseases like cholera and the Black Death resulted from "miasma" or bad air. This theory was eventually replaced by the germ theory of disease, which identified specific microorganisms as the true cause of these illnesses.

Another misconception involved stomach ulcers. For a long time, stress and spicy foods were believed to be the primary cause of these ulcers. However, this understanding was revolutionized in the 1980s when two Australian scientists discovered that the bacterium Helicobacter pylori was actually responsible for most stomach ulcers, not stress or diet.

A more recent and well-known example involves the alleged link between the MMR vaccine (measles, mumps, rubella) and autism. In 1998, a study suggested this link, leading to widespread fear and a drop in vaccination rates. However, the study was later retracted due to serious procedural errors, undisclosed financial conflicts of interest, and ethical violations. Numerous subsequent studies have consistently found no connection between the MMR vaccine and autism.

The safety of Gardasil has also been called into question. Gardasil is a vaccine and the only one given to protect against human papillomavirus (HPV) in the U.S. HPV is the most common sexually transmitted infection among women and a known cause of genital warts and cancer later in life. The FDA and CDC refute that the vaccine causes cancer, as individuals have claimed in lawsuits against Gardasil's manufacturer, and no studies have found any association between the HPV vaccine and autoimmune conditions, as plaintiffs have also alleged. Litigation is ongoing.

There has been ongoing debate and research into whether living near cellphone towers or high-voltage power lines can increase the risk of cancer. The concern arises from the fact that both cellphone towers and power lines emit low-level radiofrequency (RF) energy, a type of non-ionizing radiation.

Non-ionizing radiation is generally considered less harmful than ionizing radiation (like X-rays or radon), which has enough energy to damage DNA and potentially lead to cancer. However, the question is whether long-term exposure to low-level non-ionizing radiation can still have harmful effects.

The World Health Organization (WHO), based on the current body of scientific evidence, states that exposure to low-level RF fields, like those emitted by mobile phones and their base stations, is not harmful to human health. Similarly, many studies have found no consistent evidence that living near high-voltage power lines increases the risk of leukemia or other cancers.

However, research in this area is ongoing and evolving. The WHO's International Agency for Research on Cancer (IARC) has classified RF fields as "possibly carcinogenic to humans," based on limited evidence from human studies and less than sufficient evidence from lab studies.

In conclusion, while the current body of evidence suggests that living near cellphone towers or high-voltage power lines does not increase the risk of cancer, more research is needed to definitively answer this question.

These examples underscore the importance of rigorous scientific research and the practice of evidence-based medicine. They serve as reminders that our understanding of medical cause and effect relationships can change and evolve based on new evidence. Once debunked, however, falsehoods may linger. For example, Robert F. Kennedy, Jr.'s strident opposition to vaccines was echoed by Donald Trump, who endorsed conspiracy theories about their lack of safety.

Journalists often rely on the information and language used in scientific research studies, and they commonly use phrases like "associated with" and "linked to" when writing headlines. This can sometimes contribute to misunderstandings about scientific research and the role of causation in the findings.

The Association of Health Care Journalists' guidance on covering research studies actually aims for wording that suggests a less direct relationship. Creating headlines can be a challenging task as journalists need to strike a balance between accurately conveying the nuances of scientific research and making the information accessible and understandable to a broad audience.

Any discussion of causation must address the crucial role of statistics in medical research. They provide a rigorous framework for inferring cause and effect relationships from observational data. However, statistics may be difficult to understand, and they can be misleading if not used appropriately.

In fact, one of the most common pitfalls in interpreting statistical results is confusing correlation with causation. Just because two variables are correlated does not mean that one causes the other. For instance, a statistical analysis might find a correlation between ice cream sales and drowning incidents. However, it would be incorrect to conclude that ice cream causes drowning. The two are correlated because both increase during the summer months.

Another key factor in interpreting statistical results is the sample size used in the study. If the sample size is small, the results may not be reliable or applicable to a larger population. For example, a study concluding a drug's effectiveness based on a sample size of ten people might produce different results when tested on a larger, more diverse group. New FDA guidance aims to increase diversity in clinical trials, ensuring that the data collected is more representative of the patients who will use the medication. This all but guarantees a different approach to the statistical analysis of results.

Visual representations of data, such as graphs and charts, can also be misleading if manipulated. For example, changing the scale of a graph can either exaggerate or minimize apparent differences, leading to misinterpretation of the data.

Selection bias is another potential issue, occurring when the sample used in a study does not accurately represent the population it is intended to represent. This can result in skewed results that may not apply to the broader population.

Lastly, confounding variables that are not accounted for in a study can affect the outcome. For example, if a study finds a correlation between coffee drinking and lung cancer but fails to consider that coffee drinkers might also be more likely to smoke, the results could be misleading.

In sum, while statistics are a critical tool in medical research used to prove causation, their use and interpretation must be done with caution to avoid these common pitfalls. Rigorous study design, peer review, and replication of results are crucial in ensuring reliability and validity in scientific research.

The phrase "lies, damned lies, and statistics" is often attributed to Mark Twain, who used it in his autobiography. However, Twain himself, credited it to British Prime Minister Benjamin Disraeli, although there's no record of Disraeli using the phrase.

The phrase suggests that statistics can be manipulated or misrepresented to support any argument, even a false one. It underscores the idea that while statistics can be powerful tools for understanding data and trends, they can also be misused to mislead or confuse individuals and demonstrate causality when none exists. The phrase serves as a cautionary reminder to critically evaluate statistical claims and to consider the source of data and analytical methods used to evaluate the data before assuming cause and effect.

3

The Real Forces That Motivate Us in Health Care

Doctors are motivated by metaphysical drivers,
just like those in many other fields.

Various metaphysical concepts—those that transcend physical explanations or rules—have influenced the field of medicine throughout history and continue to play a role today. The understanding of how mental processes can affect physical health is a key example. This is evident in the field of psychosomatic medicine, which studies the influence of psychological factors on physical conditions.

While the practice of medicine is grounded in the physical body, the motivations and values that guide physicians often transcend physicality. The drive to heal, to alleviate suffering, and to improve quality of life are fundamental motivations for many in the medical field. These are not simply biological drives, but metaphysical ones, rooted in empathy, compassion, and a commitment to service.

For instance, consider the Hippocratic oath and similar physicians' oaths, which include a commitment to the welfare of humanity. Physicians' oaths encapsulate the metaphysical drive in medicine, highlighting the ethical and moral dimensions of the profession.

Virtually every American medical student swears some kind of oath, either on entry to medical school or at graduation. Physicians declare their intentions to help those who place themselves in their care and the community at large, promising to serve humanity to the best of their ability by caring for the sick, promoting good health, and alleviating pain and suffering.

Furthermore, the practice of medicine also involves managing patients' emotional and psychological well-being, recognizing that health is more than just the absence of physical illness, and that promoting a "health" care system over a "sick" care system is a moral imperative. This holistic approach to health underscores the metaphysical aspects of medicine.

The medical profession is not unique with respect to its metaphysical underpinnings. Throughout history, many philosophers, poets, psychologists, and even sports players have noted that our fundamental motivations and drives extend beyond the mere biological. They propose that these drives are essentially metaphysical, rooted in our consciousness, spirit, or soul, transcending our physical existence.

Poets, for example, with their innate sensitivity to human emotions, have frequently explored the metaphysical aspects of life. They have probed into the depths of love, fear, ambition, and despair, suggesting that these elements, which cannot be explained by biology alone, drive human actions. For instance, the Romantic poets like William Wordsworth and Samuel Taylor Coleridge emphasized the spiritual and emotional aspects of human existence, often alluding to a deeper metaphysical reality. The Persian Sufi poet Hafez is often quoted as saying, "When all your desires are distilled, you will cast just two votes. To love more and to be happy."

Sigmund Freud often expressed the view that love and work are the cornerstones of our humanness. Freud's psychoanalytic theory acknowledges the influence of unconscious desires on human behavior, revealing a metaphysical dimension to our drives. Indeed, psychiatrists and psychologists have long recognized the importance of metaphysical drives. Carl Jung, for instance, posited the existence of a collective unconscious, a reservoir of shared human experiences that influences our behaviors and desires.

Sports players, although seemingly grounded in the physical, also acknowledge metaphysical drives. The desire to win, the will to persevere, the commitment to teamwork—these are all metaphysical drives that propel athletes to physical extremes. Michael Jordan famously said, "I've missed more than 9000 shots in my career. I've lost almost 300 games. 26 times, I've been trusted to take the game-winning shot and missed. I've failed over and over and over again in my life. And that is why I succeed." Jordan's words reflect the metaphysical aspects of sports, highlighting that it is not just physical ability but also mental strength and determination that lead to success.

Musicians, like poets, psychologists, and sports players, also delve deep into the metaphysical realm. Through their compositions and performances, musicians often express and explore profound emotions, thoughts, and experiences that transcend the physical world.

Music, as a universal language, has the power to stir the soul, evoke deep emotions, and connect people across cultures and times. This ability to touch the metaphysical aspects of human existence suggests that musicians, consciously or unconsciously, are driven by more than mere biological needs.

For instance, Ludwig van Beethoven, despite his deteriorating hearing, continued to compose music, driven by a deep-seated passion and a metaphysical desire to express himself. Similarly, modern musicians like Bob Dylan and Joni Mitchell have used their music to explore themes of love, freedom, and social justice, demonstrating a drive that goes beyond the merely physical. Carlos Santana remarked (January 28, 2024) to concert-goers at the Las Vegas House of Blues, "Be happy and have fun. Tattoo it in your psyche."

Musicians who have spoken about the spiritual or metaphysical aspects of their work often describe music as a form of meditation or a spiritual journey, suggesting that their drive to create music is deeply connected to their search for meaning, purpose, and connection. Perhaps most notable is the legendary jazz saxophonist John Coltrane, who often spoke about his music in spiritual terms. His album "A Love Supreme" is considered a spiritual masterpiece, and Coltrane himself described it as his attempt to express his gratitude to a higher power through music.

In conclusion, the field of medicine, like poetry, psychology, sports, music, and many others is shaped by metaphysical drives. Whether it is the desire to heal, the commitment to service, or the holistic understanding of health, these metaphysical aspects play a crucial role in the practice of medicine.

Abraham Maslow's famous hierarchy of needs, which depicts physiological needs, such as food, water, shelter, and sleep at the base of the pyramid, also acknowledges the importance of "love and belonging needs"—friendship, family, intimacy, and connection. While our physical needs for food, shelter, and survival are undeniable, it is the metaphysical drives—the desire for love, the quest for knowledge, the will to succeed—that truly define us as human beings, including doctors. These metaphysical drives shape our actions, influence our decisions, and ultimately, determine the trajectory of our lives.

4

The "Old" Days of Medical Practice

"Those days are gone forever
Over a long time ago..."

— "Pretzel Logic," words and music by Walter Becker
and Donald Fagen (Steely Dan)

A woman in her 70s reacted to one of my online essays about the importance of narrative medicine to physicians' well-being (https://www.kevinmd.com/2024/03/the-fifth-vital-sign.html). She said, "[Doctors] can't be bothered with narration, they can barely be bothered with my finishing a full statement on what brought me into the practice that day."

It is true that doctors are bombarded with administrative requests that detract from vital time with patients (see essay 45), not least of which are computer orders, lab look-ups, and clinical summary entries. These tasks can be time-consuming and often subtract from the important time that doctors could be spending with their patients. Research has shown that doctors spend nearly two hours on administrative tasks for every hour they spend with patients. This administrative burden not only reduces the quality of care but also contributes to physician burnout. By delegating these tasks to professional assistants—medical scribes, transcriptionists, coders and billers, etc.—doctors can focus more on their primary role, i.e., patient care.

The rise of Nurse Practitioners (NPs) and Physician Assistants (PAs) has been another development in the healthcare industry aimed at easing the administrative and clinical demands of physicians. These professionals have advanced training and education that allow them to diagnose and treat patients, prescribe medications, and manage patient care, thus reducing the workload of physicians. This not only allows doctors to focus on more complex cases but also helps in addressing the physician shortages, particularly in rural and underserved areas.

Furthermore, NPs and PAs play a crucial role in preventive care, patient education, and chronic disease management. Their role has been increasingly recognized and utilized, especially under the patient-centered medical home model and team-based care approach. The coronavirus pandemic underscored the importance of these roles in delivering essential healthcare services. The rise of NPs and PAs represents a transformative shift in the healthcare paradigm, enhancing accessibility and efficiency of care.

What about population health? Have NPs and PAs contributed to the overall improvement of healthcare outcomes? Herein lies the rub, for several studies have shown otherwise, finding that NPs and PAs provide inferior care compared to physicians and increase overall costs. However, the interpretation of these findings is difficult and often depends on the context and specific criteria used to assess quality and cost-effectiveness. It is important to note that the role of NPs and PAs is not to replace physicians, but to complement their work, particularly in areas where there is a shortage of physicians.

Regarding the cost, while the use of NPs and PAs might increase certain aspects of healthcare costs, such as more frequent follow-ups or tests ordered, they may also contribute to cost savings in other areas, such as reducing the need for specialist referrals or hospital admissions.

Quality of care and cost-effectiveness in healthcare are complex issues that depend on many factors. It is crucial that each healthcare provider works within their scope of practice and collaborates effectively with others to ensure the best patient outcomes. The American Medical Association has vowed to fight "scope creep," or nonphysicians gaining expanded practice privileges. As healthcare systems continue to evolve, the roles of NPs, PAs, and other advanced practice providers will likely continue to be refined to optimize patient care and resource utilization.

The preceding discussion underscores how the practice of medicine has changed over time. In the "old" days of medical practice, care was largely delivered by individual physicians, often in solo practices. Physicians were responsible for all aspects of patient care, from diagnosis and treatment to follow-up and administrative tasks. However, as medicine has become more complex with advances in medical knowledge and technology, it has become increasingly challenging for one person to manage all aspects of care.

Enter investor or equity-owned healthcare practices. This model has become increasingly prevalent in recent years as many healthcare providers seek to navigate the financial and administrative challenges of modern health care.

On one hand, investor ownership can provide practices with the capital needed to invest in advanced technology, infrastructure, and staff training, potentially improving the quality and efficiency of care. It can also help with back-office tasks, allowing physicians to focus more on patient care.

On the other hand, there are concerns that investor ownership may prioritize profit over patient care, leading to increased costs or decreased quality. For instance, practices may be pressured to see more patients, order more tests, or perform more procedures to generate revenue. Additionally, decisions about patient care could be influenced by individuals without medical training. Nearly half of private equity-owned physician practices are resold within three years—to other private equity firms—creating a "buy to sell" mentality that may not result in any long-term benefits for physician practices and their patients.

Furthermore, the consolidation of practices under investor ownership can reduce competition, potentially leading to higher prices for patients and insurers. Thus, while investor/equity-owned practices can bring benefits, it is crucial to ensure that these arrangements are carefully regulated to prioritize patient care. Both the U.S. Department of Justice and Federal Trade Commission— the two federal agencies primarily responsible for enforcing the U.S. antitrust laws—have publicly pronounced that private equity investment and acquisitions are a top priority for the agencies and are setting their sights on health care.

Approximately three-quarters of the U.S. physician workforce are now employed. The "old" days of medical practice may have had their merits, such as the close doctor-patient relationships and the continuity of care, but the rise of investor-owned practices coupled with an over-reliance on physician extenders has all but destroyed private practice and perhaps the integrity of the medical profession— and there simply is no going back.

Pretzel logic—twisted reasoning—has won out.

5

"Get Over" Toxic Situations by Leaving Them

Don't wait until hell freezes over.

"Get Over It" is a 1994 album track that marked the reunion of the Eagles after a 14-year hiatus. The tune reached number 31 on the Billboard Hot 100 chart.

The song was written by band members Don Henley and Glenn Frey (1948-2016). Henley is known for his biting, often cynical lyrics, and "Get Over It" is no exception. The song is a commentary on the "victim mentality" that the songwriters felt was prevalent in society, particularly in the U.S., at the time. It criticizes people who blame others for their problems, refuse to take responsibility for their actions, and constantly complain about their lives.

The song's message was controversial and some listeners found it harsh, but it accurately reflected the band's attitude of tough love towards those who wallow in self-pity instead of striving to improve their situations. At the risk of sounding unsympathetic to my colleagues, I believe the song's energetic anthem can also serve as a reminder to physicians to stop dwelling on negativity and start taking control of their lives.

It is clear that medical training has inculcated toxic beliefs in physicians, and physicians have been exposed to toxic work conditions. In relation to the former, physician coach Chelsea Turgeon, MD, wrote, "[D]uring our medical training, we are indoctrinated with

19

a set of harmful beliefs about what it means to be a doctor. These beliefs harm not only us as individual physicians but the profession as a whole."

Turgeon cited the following myths that are perpetuated by medical training:

1. **"Medicine is a 'calling.'"** This mantra resonates with many of us, but it is not an invitation for physicians to be exploited.

2. **"You're either in the hospital or you're in the hospital."** What, no work-life balance!

3. **"It's going to get better when ____."** Face it, even after we conquer certain milestones (e.g., passing all steps of the USMLE, completing residency and fellowship, obtaining board certification, etc.), there will always be other challenges lurking, imploring us to embrace them.

4. **"It's not about the money."** That's a true statement for most physicians, but there is no shame in wanting to be adequately compensated for our time, especially to begin paying back hundreds of thousands of dollars in student loans.

There are certainly more myths—ones that highlight unrealistic expectations of ourselves, the infallibility of authority figures, and the suppression of our emotions. However, it is precisely when we feel the need to speak out and voice our displeasure that we are told to "get over it."

Ellen D. Feld, MD, a clinical professor and medical director of the physician assistant program at Drexel University in Philadelphia, Pennsylvania, wrote, "Any traumatic experience can have lasting psychological effects, and medical education is no exception. But these effects can be overcome. It is possible to 'get over it...'" To put Dr. Feld's words into proper context, she was talking about overcoming resistance to donating organs to medical science. Still, we never can completely "get over" traumatic experiences, including medical school.

When I said that physicians should take charge of their lives, what I really had in mind was walking away from toxic work cultures and starting anew or leaving practice for a nonclinical job. I was not deluded by thoughts that physicians—individually or collectively— could change the healthcare system, which in reality is a sick care system. As I discussed in the previous essay, investors seem to be calling the shots these days.

A colleague was recently terminated from his hospital job of 20+ years. He was crushed. He quickly found work elsewhere and wrote, "Sadly, in hindsight, I finally now realize the toxic and malignant culture I have worked under and dealt with for many years. My firing may have been a blessing in disguise."

A primary care physician left her job after the hospital administration made unreasonable demands. The email letter she received was posted online and read widely. Here is the list of demands made by the hospital administrator:

- Work 8 hours per day (or more if you take time off for lunch).
- Use downtime to complete paperwork and notes.
- Refer patients to specialists whenever possible
- Schedule 32 patients per day and see at least 20 to 24
- Schedule follow-up visits as frequently as possible
- See patients the same day or next day
- Leave a morning slot open to see patients referred from the emergency department

My reaction upon reading the letter was: Why would anyone tolerate working under such conditions? How was a "suit" anointed with so much power? What does it say about the turncoat chief medical officer who sanctioned the email? This letter unmistakably identifies the reasons physicians burn out and leave practice: unreasonable demands, loss of control, time pressure, depersonalization, and others. Yet we stay in toxic situations—mainly at work and in relationships—for all sorts of psychological, emotional, or situational reasons.

Walking away can often be the most effective way to break free from a toxic situation. Leaving can be challenging, but it's crucial for personal well-being. This step requires courage and strength because it often means leaving behind a familiar environment, even if it's harmful. It is critical to remember that walking away isn't a sign of weakness or defeat, but a powerful choice to prioritize your own mental, emotional, and physical health.

The physician hosting the website where this letter initially appeared had some good suggestions for remedying the situation, such as urging Congress to step up and ease physician shortages by expanding training options, providing greater student loan support and forgiveness, and creating alternative pathways to licensure for international medical graduates.

She also suggested that State legislators introduce reforms to reduce administrative burdens. How about outlawing private equity groups from taking over hospitals and medical practices?

I was most in favor of her suggestion to fire the CEO and chief medical officer who concocted this offensive and insulting letter. Their actions were not impulsive; rather, their intentions were malevolent and bottom-line oriented—cha-ching, cha-ching.

Many years ago, I was called to the hospital auditorium to meet the new CEO of the health system. At the end of his speech, he said to the medical staff, "Don't cross me or you will live to regret it."

Everyone was stunned. I got over it. I left the organization shortly afterward.

The Eagles were never able to get over their internecine war. They tried to make amends through reunion and farewell tours but realized they would only become friends when "hell freezes over." "Get Over It" was the group's last top 40 hit in the U.S.

6

Life-Saving Impact of Career Changes for Doctors

Take control of your career by becoming the CEO of your own company—a "company of one."

A physician messaged me. He wrote he had left his job and started his own business as an entrepreneur and administrator of medical clinics. The doctor's pulse rate had decreased to 75 beats per minute since leaving practice a year ago. He wrote that his normal pulse was "objective proof" that his new career had improved his well-being. He said it was further evidence that burned out physicians should consider a career change because it just might save their lives.

Doctors, like many professionals in the healthcare industry, often face high levels of stress, extended working hours, and emotional fatigue. This challenging environment can lead not only to burnout but a range of physical and mental health issues including heart disease, diabetes, and depression. By moving into a less stressful career, physicians can mitigate these risks and improve their physical health. In this context, a career change can indeed turn out to be a life-saving decision for many doctors.

A shift in career can provide physicians with a much-needed escape from the intense pressure of clinical practice. Not all doctors find complete satisfaction in clinical practice. Some might find more fulfillment in other areas of healthcare or related fields. Roles in public health policy or medical research, for example, could align more closely with a physician's professional interests and provide a sense of accomplishment. Transitioning into roles such as healthcare consulting, medical writing, or teaching could offer a more balanced lifestyle, significantly reducing the risk of burnout.

Moreover, a new career can also offer doctors a more regular work schedule. This change can afford them more time to spend with their families and pursue personal interests, leading to improved mental health and overall well-being. A career change can offer opportunities for personal growth and the development of new skills. This can lead to increased self-confidence and a renewed passion for their work.

Tod Stillson, MD, is a practicing family medicine physician and author of the book *Doctor Incorporated: Stop the Insanity of Traditional Employment and Preserve Your Professional Autonomy.* He wrote the book with conviction that physicians are undervalued, micromanaged, and overworked. His goal was to help them discover exciting, lucrative career options and in doing so refute the binary myth that doctors can only vacillate between employment (e.g., within a hospital or health care institution) and private practice.

Doctors have more than two choices, and Stillson's employment model enables them to increase their income while enjoying more freedom and employment alternatives, both clinical and nonclinical. Stillson claims that Financial Independence and Retiring Early (FIRE) are within reach, in addition to greater professional fulfillment.

The secret to FIRE is to adopt a model whereby you can form your own small business while continuing to serve your interests, whether practicing medicine in a traditional sense, or not. Key characteristics of Stillson's professional micro-corporation model include minimal overhead, technology-enabled platforms (e.g., telehealth), location independence, and competitive earning potential through multiple income channels—a combination of employed (W-2) and self-employed (1099) jobs—known as "job stacking."

My own career pathway attests to the power of the professional micro-corporation. The first half of my career was spent in clinical care. The second half was divided between working in the pharmaceutical and health insurance industries. Through it all, I acted as a "company of one," a term coined by business professor Ronald N. Yeaple in his book *The Success Principle*. A "company of one" is similar in concept to Stillson's micro-corporation.

Acting as a "company of one" is a natural outgrowth of forming a micro-corporation. It means you are in complete control of your decisions, guided by your "board of mentors." Your direct reports are your core competencies gleaned through years of experience and education. These typically include leading, communicating, managing relationships, negotiating, and planning and organizing events. Your core competencies make you much more valuable to individuals and organizations who would potentially benefit from your services.

To cope with today's turbulent job market, you must learn to think of yourself as the CEO of a "company of one"—yourself. By becoming the CEO of your own company, you can turbocharge your career and take it in limitless directions. While a career change can pose its own challenges, it can also offer you a fresh perspective and a chance to explore new professional interests—not to mention a healthier lifestyle.

The decision to embark on a company of one or form a micro-corporation requires a strong mindset and careful consideration, taking into account your circumstances, interests, and long-term career goals. It also requires preparation, commitment, and hard work. But you can do it, and, believe me, it is worth it.

7

Alcoholics Anonymous? How About Storytellers Anonymous?

A novel idea set to real-life, real-time storytelling.

The Concept

I'd like to propose the concept of "storytellers anonymous" (SA) in medicine. Modeled after alcoholics anonymous (AA), SA holds enormous potential as a therapeutical modality, particularly for medically traumatized individuals reluctant to come forward with their stories. I want to be clear. I did not originate the concept of medical storytelling. It has been around for ages and used recently to advocate for the well-being of healthcare professionals and patients harmed by medical and psychiatric treatment. But to my knowledge, with few exceptions, *anonymous* storytelling has never been applied in a medical context. (The exception is Dr. H. Anonymous, a gay psychiatrist forced to hide his identity from the American Psychiatric Association to advocate for LGBTQ+ rights.)

Medical trauma, whether suffered directly at the hands of a medical provider or health system, or indirectly through vicarious exposure, has been estimated to account for as much as 5% of all instances of traumatic event exposure worldwide. Medically-related traumatic events are among the top five most common types of traumatic events, along with witnessing death or serious injury, the unexpected death of a loved one, being mugged or assaulted, and being in a life-threatening automobile accident.

As I imagine it, SA can provide therapeutic relief for traumatized patients though mechanisms similar to AA—by offering a supportive and non-judgmental environment for telling stories steeped in the human tradition of sharing experiences and emotions. SA could be a platform for individuals to anonymously recount their personal trauma narratives, a cathartic process that offers a unique form of therapy for patients who have been the victims of medical trauma.

The anonymity, in this context, provides a safe space free from judgment or backlash, allowing the storyteller to express their most vulnerable experiences without fear. Anonymous storytelling can provide numerous other benefits, such as freedom of expression, protection of privacy, empowerment, promotion of understanding, reduction of stigma, potential for greater impact, and fostering a sense of community.

Medicine, at its core, is a human endeavor, and the experiences of patients are rich narratives that often go untold. There is a certain power in storytelling, an ability to heal, to connect, and to educate. For those who have been through medical trauma, the act of sharing their story can serve as a form of psychological and emotional release.

Applying the concept of Storytellers Anonymous in a clinical setting could potentially revolutionize patient care, particularly in the realm of mental health. It could offer a medium for patients to share their experiences and triumphs, bridging the often-vast gap between healthcare providers and patients. By fostering a culture of shared narratives, healthcare professionals can gain a deeper understanding of the patient's perspective, thus enhancing empathy and compassion in care.

Moreover, these stories could serve as a learning resource for physicians and medical students, offering real-life insights into the patient experience of illness and treatment. They could also provide solace to other patients going through similar experiences, creating a community of shared understanding and mutual support. However, the implementation of Storytellers Anonymous within healthcare would require careful consideration of privacy and ethical issues, ensuring that these stories remain anonymous and are shared with respect, dignity, and permission.

The Setting

Selecting an appropriate venue for Storytellers Anonymous meetings would involve a careful consideration of accessibility, privacy, comfort, and the creation of a welcoming atmosphere. Community centers often serve as accessible and welcoming venues, providing rooms for group meetings and fostering a sense of community engagement. In fact, the use of community centers for AA meetings followed soon after AA was established in 1935.

Libraries can also be a good choice, offering quiet, comfortable environments suitable for sharing and listening. They often have private rooms specifically intended for community events and group meetings.

Another option could be health clinics or hospitals that have meeting rooms. Being within the healthcare setting could make it convenient for both patients and healthcare professionals. Nonetheless, to maintain participant comfort, it would be crucial to ensure that a healthcare environment is not "triggering" to patients and that meetings do not feel overly clinical.

In this digital era, online platforms have gained popularity for hosting virtual meetings. These platforms can ensure accessibility for those with mobility issues or those living in remote areas, while also providing an added layer of anonymity.

Outdoor spaces, such as quiet parks or gardens, can offer serene, natural settings for meetings, given favorable weather. The calming effects of nature can be particularly therapeutic.

Wellness centers, dedicated to promoting health and well-being, also often offer private rooms for group meetings. They can provide a calm, peaceful environment conducive to open discussions. Regardless of the venue, it would be paramount to ensure it is a safe, neutral, and comfortable space that respects the privacy and anonymity of all participants.

The Facilitator

A facilitator for SA meetings would be a prerequisite. A facilitator can provide structure to the discussion, ensure everyone has an opportunity to speak, uphold decorum, and offer support when necessary.

A good facilitator should possess several key qualities. Empathy is crucial, as they should be capable of understanding and sharing the feelings of others to create a supportive and understanding environment. Active listening skills are also important; a facilitator should attentively listen to each person's story, demonstrating genuine interest and respect.

Effective communication skills are necessary for guiding the conversation and ensuring that everyone has an opportunity to speak while maintaining a respectful and inclusive environment. The facilitator must also have a deep respect for confidentiality, upholding the principles of anonymity and the privacy of the stories shared.

Patience is another important quality, especially when dealing with emotionally charged situations. Conflict resolution skills are also necessary to manage any disagreements or conflicts that may arise during the meetings.

In terms of qualifications, a background in psychology, counseling, social work, or a similar field would be beneficial. Professionals in these fields are typically trained in handling sensitive conversations and providing emotional support. However, a facilitator could also be someone who has undergone similar experiences to the group members, as they might have a unique understanding of the group's needs. Regardless of their background, facilitators should receive sufficient training to manage the group effectively and ethically.

In essence, Storytellers Anonymous could be a powerful tool in the healing process for patients who have been medically traumatized. By giving them a voice, it allows for the acknowledgment of their experiences, fostering resilience and offering a sense of collective healing. It emphasizes the human side of medicine, reminding us that every patient has a story waiting to be told, this personal sharing improving how medicine is practiced.

8

How Will You Make Your Mark on Medicine?

Whether in academia or practice, find
a way to leave your footprint.

Just as a carbon footprint measures the impact of human activities on the environment, the concept of an "academic footprint" can be used to describe the impact a physician makes in their field throughout their career.

The "academic footprint" of a physician includes the knowledge they impart, the research they conduct, the papers they publish, and the innovations they introduce. It represents their contribution to the advancement of medical science and the betterment of patient care. This footprint is not just important—it is essential—and can be made within and outside the halls of academia.

Physicians should aim to increase their academic footprint to enrich the medical field. The larger the academic footprint, the greater the influence and impact a physician has on the evolution of healthcare. The breadth and depth of this footprint can shape treatment protocols, influence healthcare policies, and inspire the next generation of physicians.

However, some physicians have a limited academic footprint. In the case of hospitalists, for example, one study found that among 1,554 academic hospital medicine faculty from 25 academic medical centers, only 42 (2.7%) were full professors and 140 (9%) were associate professors. The number of publications per academic hospital medicine faculty was noticeably low, with a mean of 6.3, and more than half (51%) had no published papers. Promotion was uncommon in academic hospital medicine, which may be partially due to low rates of scholarly productivity.

Measuring the Size of a Footprint

The findings suggest that measuring a physician's academic footprint involves a variety of factors that reflect their contributions to medical science and education. One key metric is their published research, including the number of papers they've authored, the quality of the journals these papers have been published in, and the number of citations these papers receive from other researchers. This offers an indication of their contribution to advancing medical knowledge.

Altmetrics—various "alternative" indicators of how influential published works become—are widely used in medicine and other scholarly pursuits. Yet, these indicators are not without controversy. Nevertheless, statistics on the number of downloads/citations of papers and the prestige/competitiveness of journals and journal articles are frequently used to evaluate academic footprints.

Another important metric is physicians' involvement in teaching and mentorship. This includes the number of students they've instructed, the number of physicians they've mentored, and the feedback they've received in these roles.

Physicians' impact on clinical guidelines and policy can also be considered. This could be measured by their involvement in professional bodies, task forces, or committees that shape healthcare policies and clinical practices.

Innovation in patient care, such as the development of new treatment protocols or the introduction of novel technologies in a physician's practice, can also be a part of their academic footprint.

Doctors routinely make other invaluable contributions beyond clinical care and medical education (e.g., in areas of governance, medical leadership, quality improvement, and social justice advocacy). Also, physicians are increasingly disseminating their contributions via newer mediums such as social media and podcasts that arguably have a greater reach than traditional scholarship outlets. People trust their opinions, and thus their endorsements carry a considerable amount of weight.

Motivating Trainees to Leave Their "Mark"

It is important for physicians to motivate medical students and residents to leave their "mark" on medicine. Physicians can motivate trainees by leading through example, showing them the impact of leaving an academic footprint in medicine—for example, by initiating the sequential steps in the adage "see one, do one, teach one."

Physicians should emphasize the benefits of an academic footprint, such as professional growth, recognition in the medical community, and the satisfaction of advancing medicine. They can also highlight that this footprint can lead to opportunities for collaboration, influence in shaping healthcare policies, and the ability to make a difference in patient care on a larger scale.

Mentorship is another effective way for physicians to motivate students and residents. Through one-on-one mentoring, physicians can guide them in their academic pursuits, provide feedback and support, and help them navigate the challenges of medical research and education.

Lastly, physicians can foster a culture of lifelong learning and curiosity. Encouraging students and residents to ask questions, seek answers, and continually expand their knowledge will naturally lead to a greater academic footprint. This can be facilitated by creating an environment that values and rewards academic contributions, innovation, and critical thinking.

Non-Academic Settings

It should be noted that while practicing in an academic medical center can facilitate academic contributions, it is not a prerequisite for leaving an academic footprint. Activities pursued outside of academic settings can also leave a lasting imprint. Physicians in private practice, for example, can conduct clinical research, contribute to medical literature, and participate in professional organizations that influence healthcare policy. They can also mentor medical students or residents in their offices or through affiliations with medical schools. An "adjunct" appointment at my medical school alma mater has enabled me to extend my academic footprint for the past two decades.

Physicians who focus on "doctoring" are still contributing to the medical field. They are applying the latest research findings to patient care, they are often involved in the education of patients and their families, and they are contributing to the collective knowledge of patient care.

Whether a doctor chooses to be involved in academia or to focus solely on clinical practice, their work is valuable and necessary. Either way, leaving a significant footprint should be a goal for every physician, just as reducing our carbon footprint is a collective responsibility. Both are about making a positive difference—in the world and in the field of medicine.

9

It's Never Too Early to Think About Your Legacy

The most enduring riches in life are not physical possessions but rather the relationships and experiences that define our legacy.

A typical first writing assignment for journalism majors is to write their obituary. It encourages students to think deeply about their lives and careers, fostering both professional and personal development. Writing their own obituary encourages students to reflect on their lives, achievements, values, and goals. This self-reflection can foster a deeper understanding of what they consider important and how they want to be remembered.

Crafting their own life story helps students develop narrative skills. They learn how to highlight significant events, achievements, and personal qualities in a compelling way, which is essential for writing engaging and effective obituaries. More importantly, the lesson serves as an important reminder that while possessions can serve as tangible evidence of a person's life and interests, people are most often remembered by the memories they create with others, their actions, and the impact they have on people's lives.

For some students, this writing exercise may be the first time they are required to confront their own mortality. It can be a deeply moving experience, leading to a greater appreciation for life and a heightened awareness of the importance of living meaningfully. The relationships we build, the impressions we leave on others, and the ways in which we contribute to our communities often form the core of how we are remembered. Our values, characteristics, accomplishments, and even our challenges all play a significant role in our legacy.

Nevertheless, possessions can sometimes hold sentimental value and serve as a physical connection to someone who has passed away. They can also provide insights into a person's life, interests, and personality. Consider Sir Isaac Newton's alchemy work. Newton devoted considerable time to alchemy, amassing a significant collection of alchemical manuscripts and conducting numerous experiments that were archived and went unnoticed until well after his death—auctioned by Sotheby's in 1936 as the so-called "Portsmouth Papers" locked in a metal chest containing his private, hand-written papers and lab books, approximately one-third devoted to alchemy.

Newton's alchemical endeavors might be seen as an exception in the sense that they were a significant but less publicly acknowledged part of his intellectual legacy. They highlight the breadth of his interests and his application of scientific rigor to diverse fields of inquiry, even those on the fringes of accepted scientific thought of his time. Yet, even Newton's possessions typically hold meaning because of the memories and emotions associated with him, rather than their inherent value, proving that ultimately the way a person is remembered usually depends on several factors such as cultural norms, personal beliefs, and the nature of their relationships with others.

Furthermore, the way a person is remembered can change over time. As people continue to reflect on their memories and experiences, their perceptions of the deceased person can evolve. They might come to appreciate certain aspects of the person's character or life story that they hadn't noticed before, or they might reinterpret certain events in light of new information or experiences. Many brilliant people became better known for their evolving legacy rather than their initial legacy: Thomas Jefferson, Mahatma Gandhi, Marie Curie, and Andrew Carnegie, to name a few.

Interviews with celebrities and influential figures often include questions about their legacy and how they would like to be remembered. This gives them an opportunity to reflect on their values, achievements, and impact, and to express their hopes for the future. For instance, some might express the desire to be remembered for their contributions to their field, such as an actor wishing to be remembered for their performances, or a scientist for their discoveries. Others may wish to be remembered for their personal qualities, such as kindness, bravery, or resilience. Some might focus more on their impact on others, expressing the hope that they've inspired or helped people in some way (I'm in this group).

It is also worth noting that these reflections can give us insights into the person's self-perception and values. How a person wishes to be remembered can reveal a lot about what they consider important and meaningful in life.

One such example is the late basketball legend, Kobe Bryant. In an interview with ESPN, Bryant stated that he would like to be remembered as a person who was able to create stories that inspired children and families to bond together. He wished to be remembered as a person who inspired others to achieve greatness in whatever they pursued. (Joe "Jellybean" Bryant, Kobe's father, was remembered by friends and family for his warm personality and otherworldly talent. Joe also played in the National Basketball Association. He died at age 69 in 2024.)

Another example is the renowned physicist, Stephen Hawking. Despite his groundbreaking contributions to science, Hawking stated in an interview with the New Scientist that he would like to be remembered for his work on black holes and the Big Bang theory, but also as someone who has led a full life despite his debilitating disease (ALS).

The late Apple co-founder, Steve Jobs, is another example. In his famous commencement address at Stanford University, Jobs didn't explicitly state how he wanted to be remembered, but his words suggested a desire to be remembered as an innovator and someone who stayed true to his passions, even in the face of medical adversity (pancreatic cancer).

Oprah Winfrey, widely known for her influential talk show, once said in an interview that she doesn't think about her legacy, as she believes that her legacy is every life that she has touched. It is clear from this statement that she'd like to be remembered for her positive impact on individuals and communities.

These examples illustrate how individuals, regardless of their fame and wealth of possessions, have personal and unique desires for how they wish their lives to be remembered, often reflecting their values, passions, and the impact they've had on others.

While it's important to have a vision for the legacy you want to leave behind, it's equally important to acknowledge that achieving it involves factors that may be beyond your control. In Hermann Hesse's novel *Demian*, the character of Emil Sinclair, who serves as the novel's narrator, famously says, "I wanted only to try to live in accord with the promptings which came from my true self. Why was that so very difficult?"

Unforeseen circumstances, changes in society, or shifts in public opinion can all impact how our actions and contributions are perceived and remembered. Sinclair's life, for example, was shaped by forces between his individual authenticity and society's conformity—a central theme in human experience in general. Furthermore, people's interpretations and memories can vary greatly, meaning that the same actions can lead to different legacies in the minds of different people.

Focusing too much on your desired legacy can potentially lead to missed opportunities or overlooked achievements in other areas. It is possible to have a significant impact in unexpected ways, and these contributions can be just as valuable and meaningful, even if they weren't part of the original plan.

People's legacies are most obviously left on their grave stones. For this reason, a walk through a cemetery can uncover unique insights about how individuals perceived their lives and how they wanted to be perceived by other people. One of my favorite legacy statements comes from a deceased person buried in Walnut Grove Cemetery just outside of Columbus, Ohio. The following statement appears on the gravestone: "I told you I was sick."

Not uncommonly, health battles derail people's legacies and in fact substitute as their raison d'être. Therefore, while it is beneficial to have a clear idea of the legacy you want to leave, it's also important to remain flexible, open to new opportunities, and receptive to feedback. Striving to live in accordance with your values, and making a positive impact in whatever ways you can, are perhaps the most reliable ways to build a meaningful legacy.

While we can express our wishes about how we want to be remembered, it is the impressions we leave on others through our actions and relationships that will largely determine our legacy—not the physical possessions we leave behind. And it is never too early to think about your legacy, because thinking about it early in life helps you live with intention, clarity, and a sense of purpose.

The Afterword is where I consider *my* legacy.

10

Winding Down Your Career

Learn the difference between an "encore career"
and retirement and how to plan for the latter.

In the midst of moving and renovating a home at age 70, I finally figured out my encore career: building Bankers Boxes. Perhaps my skills will transfer to folding pizza boxes?

This is as good a time as any to use humor, i.e., while winding down your career. Most people glumly retire. It has to be done with a modicum of planning and foresight, and also joy and humor. The second-best advice I ever received was to retire when you are completely free from debt (other than your fixed expenses). The *best* advice I ever received was not to retire but rather to retire into something.

Marc Freedman, a Yale-trained MBA, originated the term "encore career," an idea that links second acts in life to the greater good. While both an encore career and retirement recognize the changing needs and desires as one ages, they differ in their perspective towards work in the later stages of life. An encore career is about reinvention and continued contribution, while winding down is more about slowing the pace and gradually stepping back from an active professional life. I'll have a lot more to say about encore careers in the next essay.

Winding down a career, which is where I currently find myself, is typically associated with reducing work responsibilities and commitments as one approaches retirement. It often involves a gradual transition from full-time work to part-time or flexible work arrangements.

For example, a senior executive might step down from their role and take on a consultant position within the same company, working the same or fewer hours but still sharing their expertise. This is the type of arrangement I have with my current employer, a health insurance company.

If you're considering winding down your career, here are some tips:

1. **Plan Ahead**: Consider your financial situation and discuss your plans with a financial advisor to ensure a smooth transition to retirement. You want to have peace of mind that you can continue a reasonable lifestyle without earned income, living primarily off your investments.

2. **Gradual Transition**: Instead of abruptly stopping work, consider part-time, freelance, or consultant work. This allows you to maintain a professional identity while enjoying more flexibility. In winding down my career, I made sure I would have flexibility to travel and visit my children and grandchildren, including "ohana" who live in Hawaii.

3. **Mentoring**: Use your experience and knowledge to mentor younger colleagues. This can be fulfilling and ensure that your professional legacy continues. Mentoring is important to me because I have an academic background and enjoy teaching.

4. **Pursue Passions**: Use the extra time to pursue hobbies or interests that you may not have had time for during your full-time career. These are hobbies and extracurricular activities that sustain your interests and are different from a "bucket list," which aims to prioritize experiences, goals, and achievements a person wants to accomplish during their lifetime.

5. **Stay Active:** Keep yourself physically and mentally active. Engage in activities that stimulate the mind and keep the body healthy.

Here are some examples of activities that can help keep both the mind and body stimulated:

Physical Activities

- Walking or Hiking: Regular walks or hikes in nature can boost cardiovascular health and improve mood. Walking is my preferred activity.
- Yoga or Tai Chi: These activities enhance flexibility, balance, and strength while also promoting relaxation and mindfulness.
- Swimming: A low-impact exercise that is excellent for overall fitness and joint health.
- Cycling: Great for cardiovascular health and can be done outdoors or on a stationary bike.
- Strength Training: Using weights or resistance bands to maintain muscle mass and bone density.
- Gardening: Provides moderate physical activity and exposure to fresh air and sunlight.
- Dancing: Fun way to stay active, improve coordination, and socialize.

Mental Activities

- Reading: Regular reading can enhance knowledge, improve vocabulary, and stimulate the mind.
- Puzzles and Games: Crosswords, Sudoku, chess, and other brain games can improve cognitive function.
- Learning a New Skill or Hobby: Taking up activities like painting, knitting, playing a musical instrument, or cooking can keep the mind engaged.

- Taking Classes: Enroll in local community college courses or online classes in subjects of interest to keep learning. As my passion for writing deepened, I enrolled in a narrative healthcare program at a local university and subsequently assisted in teaching.
- Volunteering: Engaging in volunteer work can provide a sense of purpose and opportunities for social interaction.
- Traveling: Exploring new places can provide mental stimulation and new experiences.
- Writing: Keeping a journal, writing memoirs, or starting (or contributing) to a blog can be mentally stimulating and creatively fulfilling.

Social Activities

- Joining Clubs or Groups: Participate in book clubs, hobby groups, or fitness classes to stay socially active.
- Attending Social Events: Regularly attend community events, concerts, theater productions, or local fairs.
- Connecting with Friends and Family: Maintain strong social ties through regular meetups, phone calls, or video chats.

Mind-Body Activities

- Meditation and Mindfulness: Practices that can reduce stress and improve mental clarity.
- Practicing Gratitude: Showing appreciation and keeping a gratitude journal to focus on positive aspects of life.
- Engaging in Creative Arts: Activities like painting, drawing, or sculpture that involve both mental focus and physical activity.

By incorporating a variety of these activities into your routine, you can stay active and engaged, promoting overall well-being as you transition into a new phase of life. Consider moving to a 55+ community with many of the aforementioned activities built in.

Remember, the process of winding down your career should be personal and tailored to your specific needs and circumstances. It's about making the transition to the next phase of life as fulfilling and enriching as possible, even if that entails folding pizza boxes!

11

So, You Left Practice for an Encore Career!

Healthcare practitioners considering an encore career have a variety of options to leverage their medical and non-medical skills.

As I mentioned in the previous essay, March Freedman's groundbreaking book *Encore: Finding Work that Matters in the Second Half of Life* is an insightful and inspiring account showing how individuals, particularly those in the midlife or post-retirement stage, can seek meaningful and purpose-driven work. This book offers a refreshing perspective on aging, retirement, and work, challenging the traditional notion that life after retirement should be solely about leisure and relaxation.

Freedman, a social entrepreneur and CEO of Encore.org, uses real-life stories and examples to illustrate how individuals are reinventing themselves in the second half of their lives. He introduces readers to a multitude of people who have transitioned from their primary careers to what he calls "encore careers"—roles that combine personal meaning, continued income, and social impact. Freedman presents a compelling argument for why society should not only accept but also encourage this trend. He discusses the immense potential that these individuals bring to the table in terms of experience, skills, and wisdom.

Freedman also provides practical advice for those seeking to make this transition. He discusses the challenges that one may face, such as financial insecurity or lack of direction, and offers strategies to overcome these barriers. He argues for a shift in societal norms and structures, such as flexible work arrangements and lifelong learning opportunities, to support this growing movement. Above all, *Encore* challenges conventional wisdom about aging and retirement by redefining the traditional notion of retirement from one of leisure to one of continued purpose and contribution.

The concept of encore careers can be particularly appealing to healthcare professionals. Several factors have been driving doctors and other healthcare professionals away from practice in recent years—for example burnout, administrative harm (see essay 45), loss of autonomy, violence and safety concerns, technological challenges, insurance and malpractice costs, and inadequate support systems. Regardless of the forces driving healthcare professionals from practice, encore careers offer an attractive and fulfilling pathway that allows them to continue using their skills and experience in meaningful ways.

For example, a doctor might transition into public health advocacy, focusing on preventive care and health education. They could use their medical knowledge to influence health policies, address health disparities, or drive community health initiatives. Similarly, a nurse might move into healthcare consulting, using their hands-on experience to advise healthcare organizations on improving patient care. Alternatively, they might choose to teach, shaping the next generation of nurses.

Healthcare professionals might also find encore careers outside the healthcare sector. They might move into sectors like social work, counseling, nonprofit management, or even start their own businesses. The key is leveraging their skills, experiences, and passions in ways that provide personal satisfaction and social impact.

For physicians looking to pivot into non-medically related encore careers, the possibilities are vast. While their medical training and experience are invaluable, physicians also acquire an array of transferrable skills throughout their careers that can be applied in various fields. These skills can include problem-solving, leadership, communication, organization, and critical thinking, among others. Physicians can leverage these skills in a number of areas.

Teaching is one such avenue. Physicians can draw upon their knowledge and experience to educate others in diverse contexts. This could range from teaching science in high schools, becoming university professors in subjects such as bioethics or health policy, or offering courses on health and wellness in community centers.

Writing is another option. Physicians often have excellent communication skills which they can utilize to become medical writers. They could write books or articles for general audiences about health and wellness or venture into non-medical writing genres such as fiction, memoir, or journalism.

In the realm of business and entrepreneurship, physicians can apply their strong leadership and management skills. They could start their own business, become consultants, or assume leadership roles in healthcare startups or established corporations outside the healthcare industry.

Public speaking or motivational speaking is another potential career path. With their wealth of experience and knowledge, physicians can make compelling public or motivational speakers, providing insights on a range of topics from resilience and stress management to leadership and work-life balance.

Lastly, nonprofit work is an area where physicians can use their organizational and leadership skills to make a significant impact. They could take on management roles or become part of teams in nonprofit organizations, particularly those focused on community health or social issues.

As they consider these options, it's important for physicians to reflect on their interests, values, and passions outside of medicine. These now become the driving factors for encore careers. Seeking guidance from career counselors or coaches and networking with professionals in fields they are interested in can also be beneficial. While transitioning may require additional training or education, the result can be a rewarding encore career that fully utilizes their unique skills and experiences.

12

Identity Ch-ch-ch-changes: Navigating Medicine's Transformative Journey through Retirement

My identity underwent rapid and significant changes during residency and afterwards.

Combine Erik Erikson and David Bowie and you get: identity ch-ch-ch-changes! Just as "Changes" is seen as a manifesto of Bowie's career, predicting constant shifts in musical styles, a career in medicine similarly embodies various stages of identity formation.

I graduated from medical school on May 29, 1980. One month later, on July 1st to be exact, I began my residency in psychiatry. In the interim, I got married, went on my honeymoon, and moved from an apartment to a home using our wedding money as a down payment—at 13% interest, I might add. It was a month filled with both excitement and trepidation, passing by in a whirlwind. My identity development was accelerated during this period and afterwards.

No longer a student, I was now responsible for patient care and decision-making, which required a new level of confidence and competence. The weight of these responsibilities was both rousing and daunting, as I strived to apply my knowledge in real-world settings while continuing to learn and grow under the guidance of experienced mentors.

Simultaneously, my personal life was undergoing equally transformative changes. Getting married introduced a new dimension to my identity, as I embraced the role of a husband. This period was characterized by the joy of building a life together with my partner, but it also required balancing the demands of a rigorous residency—"on-call" every third or fourth night my first year—with the nurturing of a fledgling marriage. The honeymoon, though a brief respite, was a precious time to bond and set the foundation for our future together.

Moving to a new home added another layer of complexity. Establishing a household in a new environment required adaptability and resourcefulness. It was a period of setting up routines and creating a supportive space that could serve as a sanctuary amid the pressures of residency.

In the subsequent months and years, as I continued my residency and eventually transitioned into my role as an attending psychiatrist, my professional identity solidified. The initial exhilaration and nervousness gave way to a more profound sense of purpose and fulfillment. Each patient interaction, every challenging case, and the steady accumulation of experience contributed to my growth as a physician. The confidence that comes with mastery was hard-earned, but it reinforced my commitment to the field of psychiatry and to providing compassionate care to those who were seriously mentally ill.

Parallel to my professional journey, my identity as a husband evolved further. As my spouse and I navigated the early years of marriage, we encountered and overcame various challenges, strengthening our bond. Communication, mutual support, and shared experiences became the bedrock of our relationship.

We decided to delay starting a family until after I completed my residency, but eventually the role of fatherhood was added to my identity. The arrival of children—three under the age of three as a result of twins—brought immeasurable joy and a new set of responsibilities. Balancing the demands of a medical career with the needs of a growing family required careful time management, prioritization, and a deep well of patience and love. Fatherhood enriched my life in ways I had never anticipated, providing an additional sense of purpose and a constant source of motivation.

My wife abandoned her career in teaching to become a stay-at-home mother and raise our children. This decision was pivotal for our family, providing stability and nurturing for our growing brood, which eventually included four children. Her dedication allowed me to focus on my demanding career, knowing that our children were in loving and capable hands.

As the sole wage earner, I felt tremendous pressure to provide for our family. I worked full-time and "moonlighted" two evenings a week for extra income. The fear of becoming incapacitated through a physical or mental disability and losing my ability to support my family was a constant source of anxiety. This pressure was a double-edged sword: it motivated me to work tirelessly, but it also weighed heavily on my shoulders.

After our children graduated college and became more independent, the financial pressure lessened. My roles as a physician and father were seamlessly intertwined at this point and formed a dynamic and fulfilling life. The skills and qualities developed in one area often complemented and enhanced the other. Empathy, patience, resilience, and the ability to prioritize became invaluable in both my professional and personal spheres.

Looking back, the rapid-fire changes that began in that whirlwind month of June 1980 were just the beginning of a lifelong journey of growth and transformation. Each step, whether in the hospital or at home, contributed to the person I am today—a dedicated physician nearing retirement and a loving father and grandfather.

For younger generations reading this story, here are the main take-aways:

Realize that your identity will be shaped by numerous factors; being a physician and partner are only a couple of them. Educational and career milestones, personal growth and work experiences, adapting to societal changes, and overcoming life challenges whether they be health issues, financial struggles, or difficult cases in your practice, will likely foster resilience and build character.

Embracing change and adaptability is crucial in the life of a physician, as both professional and personal landscapes are constantly evolving. Viewing these changes as opportunities for growth can lead to a more fulfilling career and life.

Balancing work and personal life is essential, despite the challenges it presents. Making time for family and personal well-being helps prevent burnout and contributes to overall happiness and effectiveness in both spheres.

Recognizing and valuing the sacrifices and contributions of your partner is important. Mutual support and understanding strengthen relationships, especially when one partner takes on the primary caregiving role.

Financial preparedness is key. Being mindful of financial planning and savings can alleviate the pressure of being the sole wage earner and provide peace of mind.

Continuous learning and growth are fundamental in the medical field. Staying curious, seeking mentorship, and striving to improve skills and knowledge are vital for professional development.

Mentoring students or residents and contributing to the education of future medical professionals have also shaped your identity.

Developing resilience and stress management strategies is necessary to cope with the demands and pressures of the medical profession. Maintaining mental health is as important as physical health.

Cultivating empathy and compassion enhances patient care and personal relationships. These qualities are foundational to being a good physician and a supportive loved one.

Cherishing and investing in your family and support network is crucial. These relationships provide the emotional and practical support needed to navigate the challenges of a medical career.

Personal reflections and milestones, including significant birthdays, anniversaries, or personal achievements, have prompted self-reflection and growth, further defining who you are today.

Acknowledge and face fears and uncertainties, such as the possibility of disability or other setbacks. Preparing for these possibilities without letting them paralyze you can help you focus on what you can control.

Keeping a long-term outlook helps in understanding that the current challenges and pressures are part of a larger, rewarding journey. Each step contributes to professional growth, solidifies your identity, and creates personal fulfillment.

By considering these perspectives, young physicians can better navigate their own paths with greater wisdom and resilience, leading to a more balanced and rewarding life.

13

Second Opinions are No Laughing Matter

Turn to the comedic genius of Henny Youngman, the "King of the One-Liners," and begin laughing.

The practice of seeking second opinions in medicine has a long history, dating back to ancient times. The concept is deeply rooted in the ethical and professional principles of medical practice.

In ancient Greece, Hippocrates, often considered the father of modern medicine, encouraged patients to seek second opinions. He believed that a different physician might have a different perspective or alternative treatment suggestions. This practice was considered a way to confirm a diagnosis, consider a different treatment, or simply reassure a patient.

In the Middle Ages, second opinions became more formalized, especially in "teaching hospitals" where cases were often discussed among multiple doctors. This practice was intended to reduce diagnostic errors and improve patient care.

The formalized practice of seeking second opinions grew in the 20th century, especially with the advent of more complex medical procedures and treatments. In some cases, insurance companies began to require second opinions before approving certain treatments or surgeries. This was done to ensure that the proposed treatment was medically necessary and appropriate.

However, second opinions have become like runaway trains—non-stop and off course. Insurance companies now require second opinions for proposed procedures, operations, medications, lab tests, and imaging studies, among others. The American Medical Association has targeted this drill—commonly known as "concurrent review" and "preauthorization"—for elimination along with other dubious and wasteful administrative practices.

The practice of seeking second opinions has become even more common due to increasing patient empowerment and the easy accessibility of medical information online. Patients often seek second opinions to feel more confident about their diagnosis and treatment plan.

Taken to the extreme, obtaining a second opinion can become an obsession, especially if a patient believes there is something really wrong with them and the doctor appears aloof or unconcerned. The terms "doctor shopping" and "drug seeking" are used pejoratively to describe the practice of a patient requesting opinions and treatment from multiple physicians.

Doctor shopping can become dangerous when the patient visits multiple doctors to obtain prescriptions, often for controlled substances, without the doctors' knowledge of each other. This is often done with the intent to misuse or abuse prescription drugs. Doctor shopping can lead to harmful drug interactions, overdose, and addiction, and it contributes to the larger issue of prescription drug abuse.

Doctor shopping may cause physicians to become the brunt of "second opinion" jokes. This is likely due to the fact that doctors view themselves as authorities in their field, and the idea of questioning or challenging their expertise by seeking a second opinion can sometimes have a humorous element. The humor often lies in the difference between the first and second opinions, with the second one being absurdly different or unexpected. Here are a couple of well-known "second opinion" jokes:

1. A man goes to the doctor and the doctor tells him, "I have bad news and worse news. The bad news is that you have 24 hours to live." The man, shocked, asks, "What could be worse than that?" The doctor replies, "I've been trying to reach you since yesterday."

2. A patient wasn't feeling well and went to her doctor. After a thorough examination, the doctor said, "I have some good news and some bad news. The good news is that you are not a hypochondriac."

Henny Youngman (1906-1998), a famous British-born American comedian, is often linked to some of the most famous doctor jokes in the field of medicine. He performed while playing short interludes on the violin between jokes. Here are a sample:

- "I told the doctor I broke my leg in two places. He told me to quit going to those places."
- "A doctor gave a man six months to live. The man couldn't pay his bill, so he gave him another six months."
- The doctor says, "You'll live to be 60!" "I *am* 60!" "See, what did I tell you?"
- The patient says, "Doctor, it hurts when I do this." "Then don't do that!"
- "Doctor, I have a ringing in my ears." "Don't answer!"
- "I told the doctor I think my wife has pneumonia. He said, "I think you're right, but I'd like a second opinion. Bring her in so I can check."

Some audiences do not immediately catch on to the last joke. The humor here lies in the unexpected response from the doctor, who agrees with the husband's diagnosis without having seen the patient, but still wants a second opinion—his own. The joke plays with the typical expectation that a second opinion would come from a different doctor. It is a classic example of Youngman's quick wit and the kind of humor that made him a beloved figure in comedy, nicknamed the "King of the One-Liners." (His best-known one-liner was "Take my wife...please.")

Youngman loved to poke fun at psychiatrists. It seems that ridiculing psychiatrists has become a time-honored tradition couched in the fear, anxiety, or discomfort associated with mental health issues or the idea of discussing personal matters with a psychiatrist. A few of Youngman's psychiatric jokes go like this:

- "A man goes to a psychiatrist. The doctor says, "You're crazy" The man says, "I want a second opinion!" "Okay, you're ugly too!"
- A woman goes to a psychiatrist. "Nobody listens to me!" The doctor says, "Next!"
- A man walks into a psychiatrist's office. "What do you do for a living?" "I'm an auto mechanic." The psychiatrist remarks, "Get under the couch!"

One of my favorite Youngman jokes is this one: "This guy asked his doctor, 'Will I be able to play the piano after my operation?'" And the doctor says "Sure." And the guy says, "Funny, I couldn't do it before." The last laugh is on the doctor. The humor highlights an all-to-common problem between doctors and patients: doctors' unfamiliarity with their patients' personal lives.

Medical jokes in general, and "second opinion" jokes in particular, play on the unexpected, and the humor comes from the surprising twist in the doctor's opinion. It is important to remember that these are just jokes, and in real medical practice, second opinions are taken very seriously as they can be crucial in ensuring the best care for patients.

Still, I hope these jokes bought a smile to your face.

14

Publish or Perish Your Way to Tent City

Medical universities should strive to create a supportive and balanced academic environment.

I was corresponding with a good friend, a retired English teacher, who said he wasn't doing much writing these days. A few of his recent poems had been rejected for publication. My friend wrote, "It's a good thing I don't need to get paid for it [publishing]. I might be in a tent city."

My friend was obviously expressing frustration and disappointment with his lack of success in getting his poems published. His reference to "tent city," a term used to describe makeshift communities of homeless people living in tents, seemed a bit peculiar given that it is not necessary for him to make money from writing poetry—he and his wife live off of their investments and they are not destitute or facing financial hardship.

My friend was clearly referring to the "publish or perish" aphorism describing the pressure to publish scholarly work in order to succeed in an academic career. The phrase "publish or perish" highlights the pressure academics often face to continuously produce publishable material. If they don't, they risk their careers stagnating or ending (the "perish" part).

The phrase "publish or perish" originated in the context of academia almost 100 years ago, but its exact origins are unknown. In *The Academic Man: A Study in the Sociology of a Profession*, a 1942 book by sociologist Logan Wilson, there is a chapter on prestige and the research function. Wilson stated: "The prevailing pragmatism forced upon the academic group is that one must write something and get it into print. Situational imperatives dictate a 'publish or perish' credo within the ranks" (p. 197). However, it is unknown whether Wilson was citing or coining the phrase.

Nevertheless, the phrase "publish or perish" quickly gained widespread use and spread to academic environments worldwide. It has been both criticized and defended. Critics say it promotes quantity over quality and can lead to stress and burnout. Supporters argue that it encourages productivity and maintains a high standard of research. Regardless of these debates, the phrase "publish or perish" remains well-grounded in the lexicon and is a reality in many academic fields, including medicine.

Medical faculty members are often required to produce a significant amount of scholarly work. This includes research papers, articles, and studies published in peer-reviewed medical and scientific journals. The pressure to publish in medicine is driven by several factors. Career advancement is often tied to the quantity and quality of published work. Professors who publish regularly are more likely to receive promotions, tenure, and salary increases, although the publish or perish culture might also perpetuate gender and racial bias in academic institutions.

The reputation of a medical university is also linked to the research output of its faculty, with higher publication rates often leading to better rankings. This, in turn, attracts more funding and higher quality students.

Funding is another key driver of the "publish or perish" culture. Many grant agencies require evidence of productivity in the form of publications, so medical researchers are under pressure to publish to secure future funding. Additionally, publishing research findings is an essential part of scientific progress, allowing for the dissemination of knowledge, advances in medical science, and improvements in patient care.

However, the pressure to publish can also have negative implications. It can compromise the quality of research and lead to scientific misconduct as researchers rush the process or cut corners to meet publication demands. It can also discourage innovative but risky research projects that may not result in immediate publications. The constant pressure can also deter potential academics from pursuing a career in medical research.

The "publish or perish" culture affects both physician and non-physician faculty members in medical universities, but the impact and expectations can differ based on their roles and responsibilities.

Physicians in academic settings often have three roles: provide clinical care, teach medical students and residents, and conduct research. The pressure to publish for these physicians can be intense, as they must balance their time between patient care, teaching, administrative duties, and research. However, their clinical experiences can provide valuable insights and data for research, and their publications often focus on clinical studies and case reports that directly impact patient care. Some physicians gravitate toward clinical trials to determine the efficacy of drugs and devices.

On the other hand, non-physician faculty members, such as medical researchers or educators, may have more time dedicated to research as it is a major part of their job description. They are often expected to consistently produce research and may have more pressure to secure grant funding, which often depends on their publication record. Their research often spans basic sciences, medical education, or public health issues.

However, it is important to note that the "publish or perish" culture can lead to stress and burnout in both groups. Balancing the demands of clinical work, teaching, and research can be challenging for physician faculty, while non-physician faculty may face intense competition for grants and pressure to publish. Medical universities should therefore consider these unique pressures and work towards creating a supportive environment that values both quality and quantity in academic output.

Medical universities can take several steps in this regard. For instance, they can provide faculty with resources and training to improve their research and writing skills. This could include workshops on research methodology, statistical analysis, and scientific writing, which would help faculty produce high-quality research.

Mentorship programs can also be beneficial. Pairing junior faculty with experienced researchers can provide them with guidance and support as they navigate the academic landscape. These mentors can share their knowledge and experience, helping their mentees avoid common pitfalls and succeed in their academic endeavors.

Additionally, universities can encourage collaboration among faculty. Research is often a team effort, and fostering a collaborative rather than competitive ("cut-throat") culture can lead to more impactful and higher quality research. This can also help distribute the research burden among several individuals, reducing the pressure on any single person.

In terms of assessing academic output, universities can move away from solely counting the number of publications. Instead, they can also consider the quality of the research, its impact on the field, and the faculty member's contribution to the research team. "One brilliant article should outweigh one mediocre book," noted cultural critic Camille Paglia.

Lastly, providing support for grant writing can also be helpful. Securing funding is a significant part of academic research and can be a major source of stress. Offering resources and assistance with grant writing can increase the chances of success and reduce the pressure on faculty.

These strategies can help medical universities create a more supportive and balanced academic environment, reducing the negative impacts of the "publish or perish" culture. It is crucial for medical universities to achieve this balance to ensure the well-being of their faculty.

15

Appreciate the People in Your Life

Little words can make a big difference.

One of my all-time favorite quotes from the original Star Trek episodes ("Balance of Terror") is spoken by Dr. McCoy to Captain Kirk: "In this galaxy, there's a mathematical probability of three million Earth-type planets. And in all of the universe, three million million galaxies like this. And in all of that, and perhaps more, only one of each of us... [pause]...Don't destroy the one named Kirk."

McCoy is waxing philosophic. He's saying that despite the enormous vastness of the universe, there is only one of you. You are unique and quite irreplaceable. So don't destroy yourself. (Kirk was about to wage battle with the Romulans). And while three million million must have seemed like a large number in 1966, it turns out he may have been off by about three orders of magnitude.

Nevertheless, the message hits home: everyone is special, more specifically, that Kirk was special to McCoy. I ask, who is special in your life—and have you told them recently how much you appreciate them?

Nowadays, it is common to hear people say "I appreciate you." I've gotten used to it, but quite frankly it unnerves me a bit and I just smile and nod dumbly not knowing if I should thank them for their special appreciation of *me* as they stare into my soul.

This expression has been popularized by the television show *Ted Lasso*, an Apple TV comedy/drama of an American football coach hired to manage a British soccer team. Ted doesn't know the sport, the rules, or much about the culture, but what he lacks in hard facts he more than makes up for in soft skills.

Ted often asks for input from others both for new ideas and to get them on board to his way of thinking. When he gets an answer that's not correct or not what he's looking for he'll say something like "that's a great idea, just not the one I'm looking for" or "I appreciate you weighing in" or "love you jumping in but nope, that's not it." All said with eye contact, softness in his face, and a light tone.

People used to say "I appreciate it" when you did something for them. I have thought that the phrase "I appreciate you" is wrong or strange, hovering somewhere between "thanks" and "I love you," but some people apparently believe that it is not only okay to use it but important to let others know that you appreciate their good deeds. If you're undecided about whether to use the phrase or aren't sure what to say, "I (really) appreciate it" may sound more normal when somebody does a favor for you.

However, there are plenty of situations where "I appreciate you" is appropriate to use. A person may say it to a spouse, partner or close friend, as a way of expressing thankfulness for that person's presence in their life. In such a situation, "I appreciate you" is not necessarily said in response to any preceding comment or act, but often just as a spontaneous and non-specific expression of emotional connection and gratefulness for the relationship.

I heard the phrase when some college students expressed their gratitude to their favorite security guard for his long service. The security guard was in charge of a dorm in a college. The students lived in the dorm. They seemed to have an emotional connection with him.

I can imagine being one of those students and saying "I appreciate you" when I mean that I feel respect and some affection for the security guard—not just for his doing the thankless and possibly dangerous job he's been doing for years—but also for the way he treats the students he sees every day. I picture him interacting with students in such a way that they recognize (maybe unconsciously) that he has their safety at heart and takes pride in protecting them.

I've been supervising a nurse practitioner for several years. She routinely says "I appreciate you" every time I give her advice on managing one of her patients. I "appreciate" her acknowledgment of my skills and abilities, but hey, I'm just doing my job. Yet, I like the way she softly intones, "I appreciate you, Dr. Lazarus," casting a slight show of affection. Maybe I'm reading too much into it. I should only interpret her acknowledgement as "I want you to know that I notice your efforts and I'm grateful."

I've observed that in many professional contexts, especially in medicine, the phrase "I appreciate you" can provide us with a powerful alternative when "thanks" may not pack enough punch. My version of the phrase usually takes into account my southern exposure: "I appreciate y'all for helping me out." When I'm back north, especially in my hometown of Philadelphia, it usually comes out as: "I appreciate youz."

Here are some examples where "I appreciate you" might be especially impactful in a medical setting:

- When acknowledging team effort: "I appreciate you for your hard work and dedication during the night shift. Your efforts made a significant difference for our patients."
- In recognizing patient care: "I appreciate you for the compassionate care you provided to Mrs. Smith. Your kindness and professionalism are truly commendable."

- When expressing gratitude to support staff: "I appreciate you for always keeping the clinic running smoothly. Your organizational skills are indispensable to our team."
- To thank colleagues for their support: "I appreciate you for covering my shift last week. Your willingness to help out is greatly valued."
- For encouraging team morale: "I appreciate you all for your continuous dedication and hard work. Together, we make a great team."
- In patient communication: "I appreciate you for trusting us with your care. Your cooperation and positivity help us provide the best possible treatment."

Using "I appreciate you" in these contexts helps to foster a positive and supportive environment, highlighting the importance of each individual's contributions and promoting a culture of mutual respect and gratitude. Adopting this phrase can help strengthen relationships, boost morale, and create more enjoyable moments.

Go on, then, sprinkle the sparkle of gratitude on your coworkers and the special people in your life. Make their day shine brighter with your words: "I appreciate you."

16

The Artificially Intelligent Physician

Envisioning the role of an AI doctor from sci-fi
accounts is intriguing, if not alarming.

WarGames is a 1983 American Cold War science fiction film directed by the legendary John Badham. The film's premise revolves around a young computer whiz kid named David Lightman (Matthew Broderick) who accidentally connects to a top-secret supercomputer which has complete control over the U.S. nuclear arsenal. The supercomputer, named WOPR (War Operation Plan Response), is designed to predict possible outcomes of nuclear war. Mistaking the computer's simulation for a real-life game, David starts playing a nuclear war scenario, causing a national nuclear missile scare and almost starting World War III.

While the movie itself does not directly relate to the field of medicine, the themes of technology, ethics, and responsibility are highly relevant. In medicine, the increasing use of artificial intelligence (AI) and machine learning brings up concerns similar to those in *WarGames* and other sci-fi movies like *Star Trek*. For instance, the potential for miscommunication or misinterpretation of data, the ethical implications of machine decision-making, and the importance of human oversight and understanding of complex systems are all pertinent issues in today's medical field. Sci-fi movies can often serve as metaphors for the potential risks and unintended consequences of relying heavily on advanced technology in sensitive areas such as healthcare.

The Potential of AI in Healthcare

The integration of AI in healthcare is rapidly advancing. AI has the potential to revolutionize many aspects of patient care, as well as administrative tasks within the healthcare system. This includes, but is not limited to, AI algorithms for diagnosing diseases, predictive analytics for patient outcomes, automation of routine tasks, and personalized medicine based on individual genetic makeup.

AI can also help physicians with decision-making, provide predictive insights, and improve accuracy in diagnosis and treatment. It can aid in treatment planning, patient monitoring, and even in surgical procedures. AI can process vast amounts of data faster and more accurately than humans, potentially leading to earlier detection of diseases and more precise treatment plans.

Should the AI Doctor Step Out of the Virtual World?

It is important to remember that AI should be seen as a tool to aid healthcare professionals, not replace them. But deep down, many of us fear the latter possibility. Perhaps one day we will create an artificially intelligent doctor who, like Professor Moriarty in *Star Trek: The Next Generation* episode "Ship in a Bottle," will clamor to leave the holodeck (a virtual reality room able to reproduce any place and person[s] one imagines).

An AI doctor practicing medicine at the patient's bedside is an interesting vision for the future of healthcare.

The concept of an AI doctor is not entirely far-fetched. We are already seeing the beginnings of this with AI systems like IBM's Watson, which can analyze a patient's medical history and suggest potential diagnoses and treatments. Additionally, there are AI-powered virtual health assistants that can interact with patients, answer their queries, and even monitor their health conditions.

In one study, the use of a microphone on a secure smartphone allowed an ambient AI scribe to transcribe—but not record—patient encounters and then use machine learning and natural-language processing to summarize the conversation's clinical content and produce a note documenting the visit. Study participants were reportedly "blown away" by the ability of the technology to appropriately filter the conversation from a transcript into a clinical note. The AI scribe saved doctors an hour at the keyboard every day.

However, while AI can analyze data and provide clinical summaries and recommendations, it is important to remember that the practice of medicine involves more than just data analysis. It requires empathy, understanding, and human connection. These factors are currently beyond the capabilities of AI. Therefore, while an AI doctor might be able to assist with clinical decisions or administrative tasks, the need for human healthcare professionals who can provide compassionate care and understand the nuances of human health and disease will always remain.

This is where the concept of creating an AI doctor from a holodeck becomes intriguing. If we could create an AI doctor that not only processes data and makes clinical decisions but also interacts with patients in a human-like manner, the potential benefits could be amazing. It could allow for 24/7 availability of medical care, decrease the burden on human doctors, and provide a consistent quality of care. The AI physician could be programmed with the most up-to-date medical knowledge and guidelines, ensuring patients receive the best possible treatment.

Lingering Questions and Concerns

However, even with this advanced technology, some challenges would remain. Ethical considerations, such as who is responsible when an AI doctor makes a mistake, would still need to be addressed. Furthermore, while a holodeck AI doctor might be able to mimic human interactions, it may still lack genuine empathy and understanding—and be no better than an android.

In one episode of *Star Trek* ("Requiem for Methuselah"), attempts to instill emotions in an android ("Rayna," played by Louise Sorel) overwhelmed her and caused her death. Future iterations of *Star Trek*, most notably *Star Trek: Voyager*, employed holographic representations of a doctor, to be used primarily in medical emergencies. The doctor is programmed to become more like people, but its attempts to build human experiences, attributes, senses, and feelings into the doctor's subroutines are often disastrous.

So, although the potential benefits of an AI doctor could be enormous, the concept should still emphasize that AI complements human healthcare professionals rather than replaces them. It is also essential to remember that the use of such technology should always be guided by the principles of medical ethics and the ultimate goal of improving patient care.

Why is it important to mention that AI should be deployed for the betterment of healthcare? Because science fiction accounts tend to portray the nefarious side of AI (think: the medical thriller *The Algorithm Will See You Now*, by Jennifer Lycette, MD). And let's not forget that Professor Moriarty actually seized control of The Enterprise and endangered the crew, demanding that Captain Picard find a way to transfer him into the real world.

Until the benefits of AI are fully realized and portrayed in a less sinister or dystopian light—which can contribute to public fear and misunderstanding—we should probably close the holodeck.

17

Balancing the Burden of Clinician Oversight of Artificial Intelligence

By prioritizing efficiency and convenience over depth of understanding and human connection, clinicians of the future risk becoming AI robots rather than compassionate healers.

Just about everything I've read about artificial intelligence (AI) concludes that AI has tremendous transformative powers due to its array of applications in medical practice, as discussed in the previous essay. At the same time, we are told that AI is not a replacement for clinicians and, in fact, requires clinician oversight to prevent inconsistencies, inaccuracies, and even "hallucinations."

Additional criticisms of AI surround its genie-like capabilities and allure. AI can quickly lead physicians, particularly trainees, to rely on it for assistance in clinical judgments and medical decision-making. There is growing concern about its abuse and its implications for the integrity of learning and, ultimately, patient care. AI may lead students to circumvent the cognitive processes involved in synthesizing information, forming hypotheses, and refining clinical reasoning—skills that are fundamental to becoming competent physicians.

Without clinical oversight from "real" doctors, there may be a hefty price to pay for the convenience of AI. Relying on answers spewed by AI may create a false sense of proficiency and hinder the cultivation of critical inquiry and self-directed learning—qualities that are indispensable in a rapidly evolving field like medicine. When AI reduces a clinician's motivation to learn deeply about topics because they already "learned" about them from a bot, there is a cause for alarm.

AI's drawbacks and potential for abuse mandate that clinicians play a role in validating AI outputs, ensuring that recommendations are accurate and aligned with the best interests of the patient. Clinicians must not let AI's efficiency and convenience substitute for the depth of understanding and human connection required to practice effectively. Clinicians must also address the ethical implications of AI use, safeguarding patient privacy and maintaining trust in the healthcare system.

Validation of AI Outputs: While AI can process vast amounts of data and identify patterns quickly, it may not always account for the complexity and variability of individual patient cases. Ultimately, clinicians are responsible for scrutinizing the recommendations and findings generated by AI systems. Clinicians must use their extensive medical knowledge and experience to interpret AI outputs, validate their accuracy, and determine their clinical relevance. They must consider the broader context of the patient's health, including comorbidities, patient history, and other nuances that AI might miss. This critical evaluation ensures that AI recommendations are not blindly followed but are integrated thoughtfully into patient care.

Ethical Oversight: The use of AI in healthcare raises important ethical considerations, including issues related to patient privacy, data security, and informed consent. Clinicians must play a pivotal role in addressing these concerns. They must ensure that AI systems are used in ways that respect patient autonomy and confidentiality. By maintaining transparency with patients about how AI is used in their care, clinicians help build and maintain trust. They also advocate for the ethical use of AI, ensuring that biases in AI algorithms are identified and mitigated, and that all patients receive equitable care.

Maintaining Patient Trust: Trust is a cornerstone of the patient-clinician relationship. As AI becomes more integrated into healthcare, clinicians must act as intermediaries who explain AI findings and recommendations to patients in understandable terms. They must reassure patients about the role of AI, emphasizing that it is a tool to support, not replace, human judgment. This communication helps patients feel more comfortable and confident in their care, knowing that their treatment is guided by both advanced technology and compassionate human oversight.

The necessary involvement of clinicians in AI operations begs the question of whether AI saves them time or adds an extra layer of burden? Again, virtually everything I've read suggests that while the medical oversight of AI does add a layer of responsibility for clinicians, it is designed to enhance, not hinder, their practice.

AI can save time in several ways, such as automating routine tasks, providing quick access to large datasets, and offering preliminary analyses that clinicians can build upon. For example, AI can streamline administrative tasks like scheduling and documentation, freeing up more time for direct patient care. As I noted in the previous essay, AI scribes show early promise in reducing the amount of time spent writing progress notes, saving doctors up to an hour of typing each day.

In diagnostics, AI can quickly analyze imaging or lab results, allowing clinicians to focus on critical decision-making rather than data processing. Using AI, radiologists in Denmark have improved breast cancer screening performance and reduced the rate of false-positive findings. Radiologists' reading workload was lowered by 33.4%.

The key to balancing the burden and benefits of AI is effective integration and collaboration. Healthcare systems need to provide adequate training for clinicians to use AI tools confidently and competently. Additionally, robust support structures, such as interdisciplinary teams that include data scientists and IT specialists, can help manage the technical aspects of AI, allowing clinicians to focus on their core medical expertise. When AI systems are well-designed and seamlessly integrated into clinical workflows, they create synergies that lead to more efficient and effective patient care.

While the oversight of AI does introduce additional responsibilities for clinicians, it is a necessary and valuable aspect of modern healthcare. By validating AI responses and addressing ethical implications, clinicians ensure that AI contributes positively to patient care. With proper integration and support, AI can ultimately save time and enhance the quality of care, allowing clinicians to leverage technology while maintaining their essential role as trusted healthcare providers.

18

Aging and Contextual Discrepancies in Displays of Strong Emotion

How the time-honored tradition of a baseball catch became a "test" for a brain injury.

I find myself becoming more passionate with age, swept into a sea of emotions during certain movie scenes, even crying during my favorite rock songs as the lyrics and melody crescendo and become one. It doesn't matter that the neural mechanisms underlying musical emotions have yet to be fully understood. Musical passages can suddenly creep up on me and make me weep, especially if it's a song I haven't heard in a while. Perhaps the emotional connection is to my youth, or to my uncertain future, cherishing a song I may not hear again in my lifetime.

What is known is that the brain has the ability to adapt and change over time, so-called neuroplasticity. This means that our emotional responses can evolve based on the kinds of experiences and stimuli we are exposed to over the years. It is not uncommon for people to experience heightened emotions as they age, and several factors have been shown to contribute to this phenomenon.

Life experiences play a significant role, as accumulating a wealth of experiences can make us more empathetic and attuned to the emotional content in movies, music, and other forms of art. These experiences can make certain scenes or songs resonate more deeply within us, unexpectedly releasing a swell of emotions that overcomes us.

Hormonal changes that come with aging can also affect emotional regulation. For instance, changes in levels of hormones like estrogen and testosterone can influence mood and emotional responses. I went so far as to ask my primary care physician to check my testosterone level (it was normal).

Psychological growth often accompanies aging, leading to a greater understanding of oneself and one's emotions. This growth can result in a deeper appreciation for the emotional subtleties in art and life.

Cognitive changes that occur with aging can affect how we process and respond to emotional stimuli. Older adults might prioritize positive emotional experiences and be more affected by emotionally charged content.

Shifts in social roles and relationships, such as becoming a grandparent, retiring, or experiencing the loss of loved ones, can also impact emotional responses, contributing to a heightened emotional state.

My emotional outbursts are few and far between, and they usually occur when I am alone. They do not cause me distress or interfere with my daily life. I am not concerned by them, but occasionally my children become alarmed (amused?) by my unexpected display of affect when I am in their presence—for example, while watching a movie. I reassure them that these are "happy" tears, an outgrowth of my finely tuned emotions, part of my physiology, and acquired with age—like a good bottle of wine that becomes richer and more complex over time, revealing unexpected and nuanced flavors that were not there in its youth.

I don't intend to make my children feel uncomfortable or think that their dad is "off his rocker." Still, several of them are healthcare professionals, and they are aware of a condition called "pseudobulbar affect."

Pseudobulbar affect (PBA) is a neurological condition that presents with sudden, uncontrollable episodes of crying or laughing, which at first blush might explain my emotional reactions. The difference is that individuals with PBA experience involuntary episodes of crying, laughing, or other emotional displays that *don't match the context*. These episodes can occur spontaneously and may not reflect the person's actual feelings.

For example, imagine a person attending a funeral or a serious meeting where the atmosphere is somber and respectful. Suddenly, they burst into uncontrollable laughter. Despite understanding the gravity of the situation and feeling the appropriate emotions of sadness or solemnity, they are unable to control their laughter. This reaction is not aligned with the expected emotional response to the context.

Consider a scenario where someone is at a celebratory event, such as a wedding or a birthday party, where everyone is happy and enjoying themselves. In the midst of the celebration, the person begins to cry uncontrollably. Even though they are not feeling sad or distressed, the tears flow without their control. This incongruous emotional display can be confusing and distressing for both the individual and those around them.

PBA is often linked to conditions or injuries that impact the brain. It can be associated with stroke, multiple sclerosis, amyotrophic lateral sclerosis, traumatic brain injury, Parkinson's disease, and Alzheimer's disease, among others. A thorough neurological examination is important to assess any of these underlying conditions and to rule out depression as a possible cause of symptoms.

While there is no cure for PBA, treatment focuses on managing the symptoms. Medications can help reduce the frequency and severity of episodes. These may include certain antidepressants and a combination of dextromethorphan and quinidine. Behavioral strategies, such as distraction methods or breathing exercises, can also be helpful in managing episodes.

For those with PBA, open communication with family members and caregivers is crucial. Educating loved ones about the condition can help them understand and respond appropriately to the episodes. Caregivers play an important role in their loved one's care team and are in a special position to help make an impact.

Every spring, I try to gather our family to watch *The Field of Dreams*, one of the greatest father and son bonding movies. Without fail, I wail at the end when Ray Kinsella (Kevin Costner) asks his dad if he wants to have a catch. At first, my wife and daughters were astonished by my reaction, Now, after a half-dozen or so family viewings, they are accustomed to it. I can see them nudging each other on the sofa, as if to say: "Wait for it. Here it comes. Dad's going to ball again!"

If there is concern that your emotional responses might be related to PBA, it would be wise to consult with a healthcare professional. They can provide a thorough evaluation and determine if further investigation or treatment is needed. This approach can help ensure that your emotional expressions are indeed a normal part of aging and not indicative of PBA or another neurological condition.

Also, if you are a father and happen to watch *The Field of Dreams* with your adult son, notice his reaction to the final scene as he, too, unabashedly wipes away his tears.

19

The Risks of Digital Health Companies to Psychiatric Patients

*A federal indictment of healthcare executives—the first of
its kind—highlights concern about tele-mental-health.*

In early 2022, in the midst of the coronavirus pandemic, I considered practicing psychiatry via telehealth. I looked into two tele-mental-health companies in particular—Cerebral and Done Global, Inc. (hereafter "Done")—and turned them both down. I did not believe their ethics measured up. In the case of Done, I asked to be withdrawn from consideration as medical director because I believed the company lacked adequate infrastructure and was exclusively focused on treating patients with ADHD.

Sure enough, on June 13, 2024, executives from Done were arrested and charged with fraud. Federal authorities alleged that the founder and clinical president (a psychiatrist) orchestrated a scheme to profit from Adderall prescriptions. DEA administrator Anne Milgram wrote, "The defendants allegedly preyed on Americans and put profits over patients by exploiting telemedicine rules that facilitated access to medications during the unprecedented COVID-19 public health emergency, instead of properly addressing medical needs, the defendants allegedly made millions of dollars by pushing addictive medications."

The Department of Justice said the indictment is the first criminal drug distribution prosecution against a telehealth company dealing in controlled substances. Done said in a statement that it "disagrees" with the charges and that both executives were "presumed innocent." Well before the indictment, *Forbes Health* commented, "It's worth noting that pharmacies across the country have started blocking or delaying prescriptions from telehealth companies (including Done) over concerns that doctors are over-prescribing ADHD medications such as Adderall."

The allegations against Done—accusing the company of arranging the prescription of over 40 million pills of Adderall and other stimulants, resulting in more than $100 million in revenue—are deeply troubling. They highlight the severe ethical and legal breaches that can occur when corporate greed potentially jeopardizes patient health and safety. The charges underscore a critical message: corporate executives prioritizing profit over patient well-being, even through technological innovations, will face accountability. Moreover, anyone believed to be exploiting patients will be prosecuted to the fullest extent of the law: Done's executives each face up to 20 years in prison if convicted.

What makes this situation particularly unsettling is that it compounds the vulnerability of psychiatric patients. In essence, telehealth adds another layer of defenselessness to an already vulnerable and stigmatized population. Psychiatric patients often require comprehensive, in-person evaluations and ongoing monitoring that can be challenging to replicate through virtual platforms. The absence of physical presence can make it difficult for healthcare providers to fully assess the nuances of a patient's mental state, potentially leading to misdiagnoses or inappropriate treatment plans.

Additionally, the reliance on digital communication tools can exacerbate feelings of isolation or anxiety in some psychiatric patients, who may struggle with the lack of personal interaction. The convenience of telehealth also raises the risk of over-prescription or inappropriate prescription of controlled substances, as it can be easier for unscrupulous providers to bypass rigorous checks and balances that are typically in place in traditional healthcare settings. This can lead to increased instances of medication misuse or abuse, further endangering these patients.

Ironically, the digital domain can cause unintended roadblocks to treatment. While it is clear that for those in remote or underserved areas, telehealth has been a game-changer, providing much-needed access to healthcare services that might otherwise be unavailable, many individuals in remote or underserved areas may lack reliable internet access or the necessary technology to engage in telehealth services effectively. This can lead to disparities in the quality of care received and may prevent some patients from accessing the help they need altogether.

Some psychiatric patients may harbor suspicions towards digital health companies and feel exploited by them. A February 2, 2023 letter to Cerebral from U.S. Senators Amy Klobuchar and Susan Collins stated, "Although your website claims that information entered on these intake forms is confidential and secure, this information is reportedly sent to advertising platforms, along with the information needed to identify users. This data is extremely personal, and it can be used to target advertisements for services that may be unnecessary or potentially harmful physically, psychologically, or emotionally."

Informed consent is equally critical as data privacy. Some companies may not provide clear information about data usage, storage, and sharing practices. This lack of transparency can result in patients inadvertently consenting to terms that do not protect their interests, leading to further exploitation.

Misleading marketing practices are also problematic. Companies might overpromise the effectiveness of treatments or technologies without sufficient scientific backing, causing patients to spend money on services that do not deliver the expected benefits. Additionally, high costs and hidden fees can burden patients financially, especially those already under financial strain. Some companies may not disclose affiliations with pharmaceutical companies or other commercial interests that influence their overall business practices.

The quality of care provided by some digital health companies may not meet professional standards. Patients might encounter poorly trained providers, inadequate follow-up, or lack of personalized care, which can lead to ineffective treatment and worsening mental health issues. Moreover, these platforms may not offer the full range of necessary services, such as crisis intervention or integrated care with other providers, limiting comprehensive treatment options.

For example, Done focuses on patients with a diagnosis of ADHD, which affects about 3% of adults, compared with major depression, which has 12-month and lifetime prevalences of 10.4% and 20.6%, respectively. Furthermore, by targeting ADHD, about 75% of the overall psychiatric population—those with depression, anxiety, schizophrenia, substance use and other disorders—are excluded from treatment.

Algorithmic bias and inequality also pose risks to psychiatric patients. Algorithms used by digital health platforms might not adequately account for cultural, racial, or socioeconomic differences, leading to unequal treatment and outcomes. Patients might become overly reliant on digital platforms, potentially neglecting other important aspects of their treatment, such as in-person therapy or community support.

To mitigate these risks, it is crucial to implement stringent regulatory measures, including thorough verification of patient identity and medical history, regular audits of telehealth practices, and enhanced training for providers on the unique challenges of delivering psychiatric care remotely. Ensuring equitable access to technology and support for those who may have difficulty using digital platforms is also essential. By addressing these vulnerabilities, we can optimize the benefits of telehealth while safeguarding the well-being of psychiatric patients.

The implications of Done's alleged criminal activities extend far beyond the immediate legal consequences for the involved parties. Done's founder says that she "cannot stop being creative." She might have over-reached in this instance.

20

Overcoming Barriers to Effective Addiction Treatment

Enhancing physicians' support, skills, cognitive capacity, and knowledge is key.

Addiction affects multiple bodily systems, and left unchecked can lead to major disease or premature death. While effective treatments for substance use disorders (SUDs) are available, only about a quarter of the nearly 49 million people with a substance use disorder in the U.S. in 2022 received treatment, according to data from the Substance Abuse and Mental Health Services Administration (SAMHSA).

Many doctors are hesitant to treat patients with SUDs, according to a 2024 review article published in *JAMA Network Open*. The most common reasons physicians fail to intervene in addiction treatment are lack of institutional support, skill, cognitive capacity, and knowledge.

Institutional support is crucial for physicians in treating addiction effectively. This support includes access to resources such as addiction specialists, counseling services, and inpatient treatment facilities, as well as policies that prioritize addiction treatment within healthcare organizations. Without these resources and supportive policies, physicians may find it challenging to allocate sufficient time and effort to addiction treatment, which can lead to inadequate care. Additionally, the lack of institutional support can contribute to physician burnout, further limiting their capacity to engage effectively with patients who require intensive addiction treatment.

Another significant barrier is the lack of skill among physicians in diagnosing, managing, and treating SUDs. Many physicians may struggle with accurately diagnosing SUDs due to a lack of practical experience and training in recognizing the signs and symptoms. Furthermore, effective addiction treatment often requires specific skills such as motivational interviewing, behavioral therapies, and medication-assisted treatment (MAT). Physicians who lack these skills may feel ill-equipped to manage SUDs, resulting in suboptimal patient care. Moreover, skilled communication is essential for building trust and encouraging patients to adhere to treatment plans, and a lack of these skills can lead to resistance or disengagement from patients.

Cognitive capacity is another critical factor. The mental bandwidth and cognitive resources necessary to manage complex cases, including those involving SUDs, can be overwhelming for physicians. Treating SUDs involves complex decision-making, such as balancing the management of co-occurring disorders, assessing the risk of relapse, and tailoring treatment plans to individual patients. Limited cognitive capacity can impair these decisions, and the high cognitive demands can lead to stress and fatigue, further diminishing a physician's ability to provide comprehensive care. Additionally, physicians often juggle numerous responsibilities, and the cognitive load of managing multiple patients with varying needs can reduce their ability to focus adequately on the intricate demands of addiction treatment.

A lack of knowledge about addiction as a medical condition is a significant barrier. Misconceptions about addiction, such as viewing it solely as a moral failing rather than a chronic medical condition, can hinder effective treatment. Physicians who are not up-to-date with the latest evidence-based practices may rely on outdated or ineffective treatment methods, missing out on advancements in addiction medicine. This lack of knowledge can stem from gaps in medical education and ongoing professional development, leading to a lack of familiarity with best practices and new treatment modalities.

Addressing these barriers requires a comprehensive approach and culture change within healthcare institutions. Healthcare organizations should invest in resources and create supportive policies that prioritize addiction treatment. Continued medical education and specialized training programs can equip physicians with the necessary skills to manage SUDs effectively. Strategies such as team-based care, adequate staffing, and support systems can help distribute the cognitive load and reduce burnout. Regular updates to medical curricula and ongoing professional development opportunities are essential to ensure physicians stay informed about the latest advances in addiction treatment.

For example, the study authors noted that most physicians involved in the treatment of SUDs practiced either general medicine, internal medicine, or family medicine in office-based settings. There is growing recognition, however, that addiction medicine in itself is a subspecialty of medicine, and rather than treat it as an add-on to practice, it should be the sole focus of practice for patients whose primary problem is addiction. Vast differences in the types of substances abused, with alcohol, opioids, and nicotine being the most common, calls for specialized expertise.

There needs to be fundamental changes in reimbursement strategies and prioritization of services for SUDs. Hospitals that do not have a focus on early care often wait for a medical crisis to intervene. That is the old medical model. As much as local, state, and federal governments are willing to provide millions of dollars for treatment and worker training, the institutions do not find it profitable to emphasize addiction treatment when cancer, heart disease and other disorders capture the attention of the population and their insurance providers.

Finally, other reasons for reluctance to treat patients with SUDs must be addressed. These most often revolve around stigma, e.g., negative social influences, negative emotions toward people who use drugs, and fear of harming the relationship with the patient by discussing substance use. As the study authors observed: "Lack of demand may also reflect stigma if it is a manifestation of unwillingness on the part of patients to seek help due to fear of social, legal, and moral judgement or a presumption by the physician that there is no addiction in their community."

Reducing stigma, although key to successful treatment of patients with SUDs, will not be enough to address the overdose epidemic and unwillingness of physicians to intervene. Physicians, themselves, must put aside any biases and act as leaders to advocate for patients with SUDs and help garner the resources to tackle this major public health concern.

21

First Impressions Count in Health Care

*By modifying our habits, we can improve
the care experience for all.*

My son, who lives in Honolulu, was enjoying his morning latte at his favorite coffee shop. He texted me and said, "The guy at the register remembered you from last year. He says you are 'super memorable!'"

"Funny," I replied, "I don't remember him!"

However, the man's remark that I am "super memorable" resonates with me. I've found that the cliché "first impressions count" holds true in most instances, especially in healthcare. These initial interactions can significantly influence how patients perceive their care and how healthcare providers remember their patients. First impressions in health care can set the tone for future interactions and relationships. They can affect a patient's comfort level, trust, and overall experience. It's a reminder of the lasting impact that even brief encounters can have on both patients and providers, as first impressions can be made within 50 milliseconds to 7 seconds.

It doesn't take a lot of effort to make a positive first impression: introduce yourself; smile and make eye contact; acknowledge concerns and provide reassurance (when possible); ask the patient whether they are comfortable; respect their time and apologize for long waits. Of course, there is more you can do to put patients at ease, but the point is that a positive first impression can foster trust, reduce anxiety, and enhance patient satisfaction.

When patients are greeted, respected, and understood from the outset, they are more likely to engage openly with their healthcare providers, adhere to medical advice, and follow through with treatment plans. This can lead to better health outcomes and a more efficient healthcare process.

In contrast, a negative first impression can create barriers to effective communication and trust. Patients who feel dismissed or undervalued may withhold important information, question the competence of their caregivers, or even avoid seeking necessary medical attention in the future. This underscores the importance of healthcare providers being empathetic, attentive, and professional from the very first encounter. Simple gestures like a warm greeting, attentive look, and clear communication can make a significant difference in how patients perceive their care.

First impressions also affect professional dynamics and relationships among healthcare workers. A positive initial interaction with colleagues can pave the way for effective teamwork, collaboration, and a supportive work environment. In healthcare settings, where multidisciplinary teams are common, the ability to quickly establish rapport and mutual respect is essential. When coworkers view each other as competent, approachable, and reliable from the start, it enhances communication, reduces misunderstandings, and promotes a cohesive team dynamic.

Conversely, a poor first impression among colleagues can lead to tension, miscommunication, and a lack of cooperation, which can ultimately affect patient care. Healthcare professionals must often make quick decisions and rely on each other's expertise, so trust and respect are paramount. By making a good first impression, healthcare workers can build strong professional relationships that contribute to a more positive, efficient, and effective workplace.

Of all the medical specialists, psychiatrists probably face the most unique challenge of making a good first impression because they must balance hospitality with professional neutrality. Maintaining neutrality is crucial for fostering an open and non-judgmental therapeutic environment, yet psychiatrists can still make a positive first impression by focusing on several key aspects of their initial interactions with patients. For example, we can demonstrate empathy and warmth, practice active listening, present ourselves as competent and professional, and create a safe and non-judgmental space for patients to "open up."

Although I have always been mindful of the need to create a good first impression with patients, the interaction I most vividly recall was anything but positive. After the initial psychotherapy session, a patient told me she would not reschedule an appointment because my plants were dying due to lack of water.

"How do you expect to take care of me?" she wanted to know.

I had no reply that could mollify her, but thereafter I vowed to pay attention to the physical environment as well as the quality of my interactions to affirm the positive first impressions I strove to create. Patients often look for signs, even subtle ones, that indicate a caregiver's reliability and attention to detail. A tidy, well-maintained office and exam room convey professionalism and care.

Doctors, nurses, and office personnel may feel that using verbal and non-verbal cues to ensure good first impressions will add time to an already busy workplace environment, or that their own personality doesn't lend itself to facilitating initial positive encounters. It is surprising how little time these communication efforts take since they focus on better, quality experiences and do not necessarily add more time. In fact, they may save time by preventing grievances from manifesting into patient complaints requiring a formal investigation and response.

In summary, making a good first impression in health care is vital not only for patient satisfaction and outcomes but also for fostering a collaborative and harmonious work environment. Whether interacting with patients or colleagues, healthcare providers should strive to demonstrate empathy, respect, and professionalism from the outset.

It's no coincidence that my 1980 medical school yearbook was dedicated to a doctor (a psychiatrist) who made the best first impression at our freshman orientation in 1976—an encounter described as "especially propitious" by our yearbook editor. Countless students sought this physician's advice and guidance. I was one of them.

22

First Impressions Count in Health Care—Part 2

Recovering from a bad first impression can be challenging but is certainly possible.

I would be remiss if I did not illustrate the significance of first impressions in health care without providing examples. Here are a few scenarios illustrating the importance of making a good first impression on patients and co-workers in various settings:

Scenario 1: First Impressions with Patients

Example 1: Positive First Impression: A new patient, Mrs. Davis, arrives at a clinic for her first appointment. The receptionist greets her warmly with a smile, checks her in efficiently, and offers her a comfortable seat while she waits. When the nurse calls her name, she introduces herself, makes eye contact, and engages in small talk to ease any anxiety Mrs. Davis might have. The doctor, Dr. Smith, enters the room, introduces himself, and listens attentively as Mrs. Davis describes her symptoms. He explains the examination process clearly and answers all her questions patiently.

Impact: Mrs. Davis feels respected, valued, and understood. She trusts Dr. Smith and the clinic staff, making her more likely to follow medical advice and return for follow-up appointments. This positive experience can lead to better health outcomes and a strong patient-provider relationship.

Example 2: Negative First Impression: Mr. Johnson arrives at the emergency department with severe abdominal pain. The triage nurse appears rushed and dismissive, barely making eye contact. After a long wait, he is seen by Dr. Lee, who seems preoccupied and doesn't take the time to thoroughly explain the diagnosis or treatment plan. Mr. Johnson leaves the hospital feeling confused and undervalued.

Impact: Mr. Johnson's negative experience may lead him to distrust the healthcare system, potentially causing him to delay seeking medical help in the future. This can result in worsening health conditions and a reluctance to follow medical advice.

Scenario 2: First Impressions with Co-Workers

Example 1: Positive First Impression: Dr. Patel, a new resident, joins a hospital team. On her first day, she introduces herself to the team members, showing genuine interest in their roles and experiences. During rounds, she listens attentively, asks thoughtful questions, and offers to help with tasks. Her approachable and respectful demeanor quickly earns the trust and respect of her colleagues.

Impact: Dr. Patel's positive first impression fosters a collaborative environment. Her colleagues feel comfortable sharing information and seeking her input, leading to better teamwork and improved patient care. Her willingness to assist also helps build a supportive and cohesive team dynamic.

Example 2: Negative First Impression: Nurse Jackson starts a new job in a busy ICU. On her first day, she appears disengaged, avoids eye contact, and doesn't introduce herself to the team. During a critical situation, she hesitates to ask for help and makes a mistake due to lack of communication.

Impact: Nurse Jackson's negative first impression creates a barrier between her and her colleagues. The team may be reluctant to rely on her or offer support, leading to potential communication breakdowns and compromised patient care. Building trust and effective teamwork becomes more challenging.

Scenario 3: First Impressions in Multidisciplinary Meetings

Example 1: Positive First Impression: During a multidisciplinary team meeting, Dr. Nguyen, a new oncologist, presents a case with clarity and confidence. She acknowledges the input of nurses, social workers, and other specialists, showing appreciation for their perspectives. Her collaborative approach and respect for each team member's expertise make a strong positive impression.

Impact: Dr. Nguyen's positive first impression encourages open communication and collaboration among the team. Her respect for colleagues' contributions promotes a culture of mutual respect and teamwork, ultimately benefiting patient care.

Example 2: Negative First Impression: In the same setting, Dr. Roberts, a new surgeon, dismisses the input of a nurse by interrupting her and downplaying her concerns. He dominates the conversation and disregards the perspectives of other team members.

Impact: Dr. Roberts' negative first impression creates tension and resentment within the team. Other members may feel undervalued and hesitant to share their insights, leading to a fragmented approach to patient care and potential oversights.

In all these scenarios, the initial interactions significantly shape the dynamics of patient-provider relationships and team collaboration. Making a good first impression can lead to trust, effective communication, and a supportive environment, while a poor first impression can result in distrust, miscommunication, and a less cohesive team.

The truth is, all of us experience a never-ending number of first impressions. They are not unique to healthcare settings.

Perhaps you visited a restaurant that was highly recommended by friends. After being seated, five or ten minutes go by without a server coming to the table. When the server finally arrives, they seem distracted with no discernible facial expression. How does this indifference make you feel?

Or what about the flight attendant who treats you like an empty seat when you try to ask a simple question? In either case, the chance for a warm, enjoyable experience is diminished after such a cold beginning.

Recovering from a bad first impression can be challenging but is certainly possible with conscious effort and time. Psychological studies suggest that first impressions are formed quickly and are difficult to change, partly due to confirmation bias, where people interpret new information in a way that confirms their initial thoughts.

One effective approach is to acknowledge the poor first impression and apologize if appropriate, showing humility and awareness. Demonstrating consistent, positive behavior over time can gradually reshape perceptions. Open communication about the initial interaction can clear misunderstandings and provide context. Seeking constructive feedback on how to improve shows a willingness to grow and adapt. Become aware of your "blind spots" by consulting a coach or counselor, if necessary.

Emphasizing your strengths and positive attributes in subsequent interactions helps build a more balanced view of your character. It's important to be patient, as changing a first impression takes time. Authentic interactions are more likely to be received positively than contrived efforts to impress. Improving communication skills and maintaining high standards of medical professionalism can further aid in counteracting a poor first impression. Additionally, paying attention to non-verbal cues like body language and eye contact can convey sincerity and respect.

Generally, many patients are open to giving healthcare providers another opportunity if the initial issue was minor or a simple misunderstanding. However, if the issue involved a serious mistake or perceived negligence, patients may be less inclined to offer a second chance. In areas with limited healthcare options, patients might be more willing to give a second chance due to necessity.

Keep in mind that everyone makes mistakes and slips up occasionally. How you address and manage these situations can not only mitigate a bad first impression but also create a lasting positive one.

23

The Ethics of Concealing Health
Issues in Public Figures

Balancing privacy and public interest are foremost.
Deception and cover ups trigger outrage and distrust.

A Balancing Act

The ethics of concealing health issues of important public figures is
a complex and multifaceted issue, involving the balancing of privacy
rights, public interest, and the potential impact on governance and
public trust. One of the primary considerations is the right to privacy.
Public figures, like all individuals, have a right to privacy concerning
their personal health. This right is protected under various laws
and ethical principles, including HIPAA and the principle of medical
confidentiality. Concealing health issues respects the dignity of the
individual, allowing them to manage their health without undue
public scrutiny or stigma. However, public figures, especially those
in positions of power, may have a diminished expectation of privacy
due to the nature of their roles and the potential impact of their
health on their professional duties involving national affairs.

Another key consideration is the public interest. Disclosure of
health issues can promote transparency, fostering public trust in
leadership. Concealment can lead to suspicion and erosion of trust if
the truth eventually emerges. The public has a right to be informed
about the health of leaders, especially if it might affect their ability
to perform their duties. This information can be crucial during

elections or in times of crisis. Conversely, disclosure might lead to unnecessary panic, speculation, or instability, which could harm public confidence and the effective functioning of governance.

The impact on governance is also a critical factor. If a leader's health issue is severe enough to impact their ability to govern, it is essential for a smooth transition of power. Concealing such issues could lead to a leadership vacuum or crisis. Public figures are accountable to their constituents, and part of this accountability includes being transparent about factors that might impair their ability to serve effectively. However, premature disclosure of health issues that do not currently impair the leader's ability to govern might lead to unnecessary political instability and could be exploited by opponents for political gain.

Ethical theories and principles provide different perspectives on this issue. From a utilitarian perspective, the decision to disclose or conceal should be based on the potential outcomes and the greatest good for the greatest number of people. If disclosure leads to better overall outcomes for society, it may be justified. From a deontological perspective, there is an inherent duty to respect the privacy and autonomy of individuals, including public figures. Concealing health issues might be ethically acceptable if it aligns with the duty to respect individual rights and confidentiality. From a virtue ethics perspective, the character and integrity of both the public figure and those making the decision are crucial. Transparent and honest communication might align with virtuous behavior, fostering trust and ethical leadership.

Contextual considerations also play a significant role. The nature of the health issue (e.g., a temporary illness vs. a chronic or terminal condition) and its direct impact on the public figure's duties should be considered. Immediate disclosure might not always be necessary or appropriate; the timing and context of the information release can significantly affect its impact. In conclusion, the ethics of concealing health issues of important public figures require a careful balancing of competing values and interests. While the right to privacy and dignity is paramount, the public's right to be informed and the potential impact on governance and public trust are also critical factors. Each situation must be evaluated on its own merits, considering the specifics of the health issue, the role of the public figure, and the broader societal context.

The President of the United States

As for the health of the president of the United States, arguably the most important public figure in the world, medical fitness carries significant implications across various domains, including national security, political stability, and public confidence. For national security, the president's health directly impacts their ability to make critical decisions, especially during crises. Any impairment can potentially jeopardize national security. Politically, the president's health can influence the stability of their administration. Prolonged illness or incapacitation may lead to uncertainty and power struggles within the government.

Public confidence is also closely tied to the health of the president. The president's health affects public trust in the government's ability to function effectively. Transparency about health issues can either bolster or undermine public confidence. Additionally, the health of the president is crucial for ensuring a smooth transition of power if necessary. Clear protocols and transparency are essential for maintaining continuity of governance.

International relations are another area where the president's health can have significant implications. Allies and adversaries alike monitor the president's health, which can affect diplomatic and strategic decisions. Economic implications are also linked to the president's health. The president's health can impact economic stability and investor confidence. Markets may react to news about the president's health, affecting economic policies and financial markets.

Finally, there are ethical and privacy considerations to take into account. Balancing the president's right to privacy with the public's right to know about their leader's health is a complex ethical issue. Transparency must be weighed against potential risks to national security and personal privacy. Understanding these implications underscores the importance of maintaining the President's health and ensuring transparent communication about any health issues.

Historical Examples

Invaluable examples from history have shed considerable light on the aforementioned issues. Franklin D. Roosevelt's presidency has long been considered one of medical deception. Americans knew he had survived polio and were vaguely aware of his restricted mobility, but they had never seen him in the wheelchair he used every day. He was always photographed from the waist up, and most people were unaware of his failing health from hypertension and heart disease until his death in 1945 from a stroke.

John F. Kennedy concealed many health woes due to Addison's disease (adrenal insufficiency), and Ronald Reagan's doctors issued misleading health updates following his assassination attempt in 1981. Grover Cleveland disappeared for four days in 1893 to have secret cancer surgery on a yacht, informing the public that he was taking a four-day fishing trip from New York to his summer home in Cape Cod. Cleveland worried that news of his diagnosis would spook Wall Street and cause a public panic, as the economy was already in a depression.

In 1972, Thomas Eagleton had to withdraw as George McGovern's presidential running mate due to his history of mental health issues. Similarly, in 1992, Paul Tsongas, a survivor of non-Hodgkin's lymphoma, encountered ongoing concerns about his health throughout his unsuccessful presidential campaign.

Donald Trump routinely downplayed the seriousness of COVID-19 and initially attempted to cover up his own infection.

Rumors swirled around Joe Biden's apparent cognitive decline (see essay 46). Multiple sclerosis, Parkinson's disease, ascending lateral sclerosis, and stroke were offered as possible explanations—without proof.

Historian David Welky, PhD, remarked that "[i]n a 24/7 news environment, where amateur sleuths analyze high-resolution video looking for evidence of weakness or blemishes, hiding ailments is far harder than it was when FDR was president. Yet, at the same time, we still encourage exactly this kind of deception by maintaining outsize expectations of perfect health."

Let's face it. No one is in perfect health. Claiming otherwise only elicits public outrage and causes further distrust of government officials.

24

Comparing Presidential Security Failures and Medical Errors

Parallels in crisis.

The breakdown in security leading to the attempted assassination of Donald Trump in July of 2024 can be compared to the multifactorial failure inherent in medical errors, as both scenarios involve complex systems where multiple layers of defense and prevention are designed to avoid catastrophic outcomes. When these layers fail, it often results from a combination of human error, systemic issues, and procedural flaws.

Both presidential security and healthcare systems are highly complex and require coordination among various components. In health care, this includes medical staff, administrative processes, and technological systems. Similarly, presidential security involves coordination among security personnel, intelligence agencies, and logistical planning. Breakdowns in all these areas were cited as probable factors leading to the assassination attempt. The fact that no agency arranged to have drones flying overhead to detect a possible threat was evidence of poor planning.

Human error can play a significant role in both security and medical failures. For instance, lapses in vigilance, miscommunication, or failure to follow protocols can contribute to both security breaches and medical errors. Earlier in the day, prior to the rally, Trump's shooter was identified at the fairgrounds. He was acting suspiciously and pacing near magnetometers. He was labeled a person of interest more than an hour before the assassination attempt. He was never pulled aside and detained by authorities to question his motives. Likewise, Trump was never asked to delay taking the stage until an all-clear sign could be given. This was an especially glaring omission in light of already ramped up security due to global threats on Trump's life in recent months.

Systemic flaws such as inadequate training, poor communication channels, and insufficient resources can lead to failures. In health care, this might manifest as understaffing or lack of proper equipment. In presidential security, it could involve gaps in intelligence or insufficient security measures. The agricultural manufacturing building used by the shooter to perpetrate his scheme was designated outside the security perimeter of metal detectors and bag searches. Why? It was very close to the field where Trump's supporters had gathered—and to Trump, himself, as he stood at the podium.

Both fields rely on a series of preventive measures designed to mitigate risks. In medicine, this includes checklists, double-check systems, and standardized procedures. In security, this involves background checks, security protocols, and surveillance systems. When these measures are not properly implemented or fail, the risk of a critical incident increases. Trump's shooter escaped surveillance and lay in waiting atop a building less than 150 yards from the podium. Yet he was confronted on the rooftop by a police officer, and Secret Service snipers had "eyes" on him for a full 6 minutes prior to the attack. Still, they waited, and the shooter managed to prevail, firing first.

The timeline was as follows:

- 5:10 Shooter was first identified as a person of interest
- 5:30 Shooter was spotted with a rangefinder
- 5:52 Shooter was spotted on the roof by Secret Service
- 6:12 Shooter fires first shots

Trump's assassination attempt was totally preventable.

Medial errors are preventable, too.

After a critical incident, whether in law enforcement or medicine, both fields conduct thorough investigations to understand the root causes and prevent future occurrences. In healthcare, this might be a morbidity and mortality (M&M) conference or a root cause analysis (RCA). In security, it could be an internal review or a congressional investigation. Both areas require constant vigilance and continuous improvement. Lessons learned from failures are used to enhance protocols, improve training, and upgrade systems to prevent future incidents. A congressional hearing and other investigations will be held to fully evaluate the incident. How long will it take before the results are known? The obvious answer is: too long.

In summary, both the failure in presidential security leading to an attempted assassination and medical errors in healthcare share similarities in their multifactorial nature, involving complex systems, human factors, systemic issues, preventive measures, root cause analysis, and continuous improvement. Understanding these parallels can help in developing better strategies to prevent such critical failures in both fields. Such strategies might include:

1. Addressing Human Factors

To mitigate human error, organizations can implement comprehensive training programs that emphasize critical thinking, situational awareness, and adherence to protocols. For instance, in health care, simulation-based training allows medical professionals to practice responding to emergency scenarios in a controlled environment, reducing the likelihood of errors in real-life situations. Similarly, security personnel can engage in regular drills and exercises that mimic potential threats, ensuring they are well-prepared to respond effectively.

2. Enhancing Communication

Keeping open lines of communication is another crucial strategy. In both fields, clear and effective communication can prevent misunderstandings and ensure that all team members are on the same page. This can be achieved through standardized communication protocols, regular briefings, and debriefings, and fostering a culture where team members feel comfortable speaking up about potential issues.

3. Transparency

Transparency is an absolute requirement in any investigation. In government and politics, transparency helps to avoid the spread of conspiracy theories. In medicine, it helps prevent cover-ups. However, statements will amount to little if they aren't followed with a change in behavior and substantive explanations that dig deep into the facts. Simply assigning blame after a tragic or near-tragic outcome does little to change the status quo.

4. Systemic Improvements

Ensuring adequate staffing levels is essential. In health care, this means having enough medical professionals to handle patient loads without compromising care quality. In security, this involves having sufficient personnel to cover all necessary posts and respond to potential threats.

5. Investing in Infrastructure and Technology

Spending in this area is crucial. For health care, this might mean equipping hospitals with the latest medical devices and electronic health records systems to streamline patient care. In security, advanced surveillance systems, secure communication channels, and modern protective equipment can enhance the ability to detect and respond to threats.

6. Preventive Measures

In medicine, checklists can ensure that all necessary steps are taken during surgeries or other medical procedures, reducing the risk of oversight. In presidential security, standardized procedures for threat assessment, access control, and emergency response can create a robust framework for protecting the president.

7. Risk Assessment and Management

Both fields can benefit from adopting proactive risk assessment techniques to identify potential vulnerabilities and address them before they lead to failures. This might involve regular audits, threat assessments, and the development of contingency plans to handle unexpected situations.

8. Continuous Improvement

Creating a culture of continuous learning involves encouraging team members to share their experiences and insights, fostering an environment where feedback is valued and acted upon. In health care, this often entails regular M&M meetings where medical professionals discuss cases and learn from each other. In security, after-action reviews following drills or actual incidents can provide valuable insights for improving protocols and responses.

By leveraging these strategies, both fields can enhance their ability to prevent critical failures and ensure better outcomes. Neither a patient's health nor a president's welfare should ever be taken for granted.

25

The Profound Aftermath of Near-Death Experiences

Did Donald Trump's brush with death really change him?

Near-death experiences (NDEs) have fascinated both the medical community and the general public due to their profound and often transformative effects on individuals. These experiences typically occur in situations where a person is close to death or facing a life-threatening condition. Common elements reported during NDEs include feelings of peace, out-of-body experiences, traveling through a tunnel, encountering a bright light, and meeting deceased loved ones or spiritual beings. The aftermath of such experiences can lead to significant psychological and spiritual changes.

Donald Trump is in the early throes of his NDE, and we have already begun to glimpse how it might have affected him in a positive way. Soon after the shooting, Trump stated he was "serene" and grateful to be alive, easing up on his usual intensity and antagonistic tone. He rewrote his acceptance speech at the Republican National Convention (RNC) to be less divisive and more unifying. However, skeptics saw this as nothing more than political manipulation, interpreting Trump's call for unity as a way to get everyone in his party unified behind him. That would mean his close encounter with death was not a conversion experience and had no transformative effect at all.

However, research shows that most NDEs do, in fact, have lasting effects, changing someone's attitudes, values, beliefs, and behavior. This is because these experiences challenge our understanding of life and death, not only leaving permanent impressions but, in most cases, experiences described as pleasant, surreal, and even glorious. Indeed, Trump's supporters appeared to have been affected by the ordeal, firmly believing that he was "saved" for a higher purpose and ordained by God (while Democrats warned he would make himself king).

However, not all NDEs are so affirming; some are deeply disturbing and upsetting. No hard evidence exists to document the frequency of frightening NDEs. The published figures vary widely, indicating that 10-20% are distressing and do not result in psychological alterations for the better. Overall, the aftermath of NDEs underscores the complexity of human consciousness and the profound impact such events can have on an individual's emotional and spiritual well-being.

A wide range of traumatic events apart from NDEs can act as catalysts for positive change, such as illness, divorce, separation, assault, bereavement, accidents, natural disasters, and terrorism. These observations have been noted for decades, broadly subsumed under the psychology of posttraumatic growth (PTG). The concept of PTG refers to the positive psychological changes that can occur as a result of struggling with highly challenging life circumstances. NDEs and other traumatic events can both act as catalysts for this type of growth. While these events vary widely, the resulting transformative effects often share common themes, e.g., a reevaluation of life priorities, a deeper appreciation for life, and a heightened sense of personal strength.

The underlying process of PTG underscores the resilience of the human spirit. Whether through the extraordinary lens of an NDE or the more common experiences of life's struggles, individuals can emerge from trauma with a renewed sense of meaning, purpose, and connection to others. This shared potential for growth highlights the remarkable capacity for personal transformation inherent in facing and overcoming life's most difficult moments.

One notable example is the case of Eben Alexander, MD, a neurosurgeon who experienced an NDE during a coma caused by bacterial meningitis. He described a journey to a place of profound beauty and peace, which he interpreted as evidence of an afterlife. This experience drastically changed his previously skeptical views on consciousness and spirituality, leading him to advocate for the study of NDEs and write about his experience in *Proof of Heaven*. Similarly, Anita Moorjani's NDE during a coma from terminal cancer led her to a full recovery and a newfound sense of purpose and spirituality, which she detailed in her book *Dying to Be Me*.

In the time since the attempted assassination of Donald Trump, he has not changed his political approach. During his lengthy and mostly unscripted speech at the RNC and in subsequent talks, Trump has continued his usual attacks on rivals without shifting away from a narrative of national decline. He continues to push his dark and dystopian political vision that will land hardest on populations whose members are already struggling. If there is a new GOP message focused on peace and understanding, it has not been prominently featured.

Donald Trump's transformation from his near-death experience has yet to occur. I doubt it ever will. His close brush with death only briefly halted the rancorous rhetoric characteristic of his first term in office. Trump admitted as much at a rally in Pennsylvania 18 days after his attempted assassination, telling the crowd, "When I got hit, everybody thought I was going to be a nice guy, and they thought I'd change. They all said Trump is going to be a nice man now. He came close to death. And I really agreed with that—for about eight hours or so."

SECTION 2

Insights

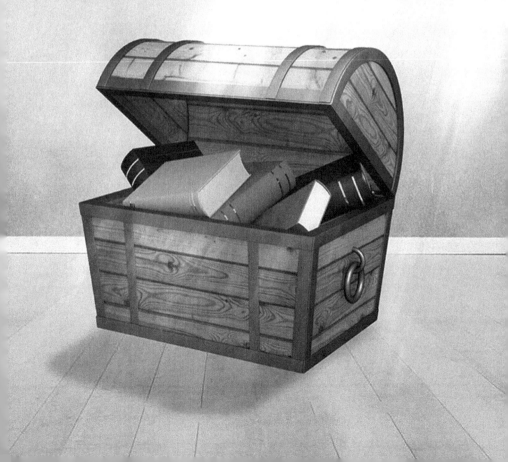

26

Star Trek and Medicine Share
Similar "Prime Directives"

Both provide a foundational ethical guideline, but
they operate in vastly different universes.

Following my evening meal, I indulged in my usual nighttime routine: I tuned into the original "Star Trek" TV series. Although I joined the episode "Return of the Archons" 15 minutes late, it wasn't a concern, given that I had watched it nearly a dozen times before. What was striking, however, was the eerie relevance it had to a discussion I had just had about creativity.

The core message of the episode explores the potential stagnation of a society that is overly conformist and lacks imagination. It underscores the importance of memory, imagination, and intuition in sparking the creative flame within a culture.

In this episode, the USS Enterprise travels to Beta III where the ship, the USS Archon, had been lost a century ago. Upon arrival, the Enterprise crew discovers a seemingly idyllic planet where its inhabitants are peaceful—even euphoric—and "of the body." In fact, the society is stuck in a perpetual state of tranquility, devoid of creativity and individuality. They are ruled by a strict and oppressive regime controlled by a mysterious figure known as Landru. It turns out that Landru is a sophisticated computer system left over by an ancient civilization that maintains peace and order through telepathy.

Captain Kirk and company learn that Landru was at one time a real person who created the computer to impose his ideals of peace and tranquility on the planet. However, over the years, the computer became corrupted and began enforcing its programming in a totalitarian manner. Kirk vehemently informs Landru that the suppression of creativity is harmful to society, resulting in the computer's self-destruction and liberation of the people from its control.

Apart from its central theme—the suppressive impact of an inflexible, regulated society on personal creativity and expression—"Return of the Archons" draws clear parallels between the "Star Trek" prime directive and the prime directive in medicine. The "Star Trek" prime directive, which forbids meddling with the organic evolution of alien civilizations, was initially introduced and elucidated in "Return of the Archons." Despite this, the prime directive was often disregarded for the welfare of the people, as seen in this episode. Captain Kirk made a compelling argument that the directive could be bypassed when a society is not alive and growing.

In medicine, we don't have the option to take life and death matters into our own hands. Our prime directive—often encapsulated in the phrase "Primum non nocere," a Latin phrase that means "First, do no harm"—asserts that medical interventions should not cause harm or suffering to patients. It is a foundational principle in the practice of medicine, guiding physicians and other healthcare providers to always consider the potential harm of any intervention or treatment before proceeding.

While both sets of prime directives operate within an ethical framework and are guiding principles for decision-making, the "Star Trek" prime directive prohibits intervention, even if it could potentially benefit another civilization. In contrast, "Primum non nocere" does not prohibit intervention and sometimes requires it, especially if the potential benefits outweigh the risks (It should be noted that throughout the "Star Trek" TV series and movies, there have been numerous instances where characters have violated the prime directive, either intentionally or unintentionally. Characters sometimes violated the directive in order to save lives, both alien and human. This often involved a moral dilemma between adhering to the directive and preventing unnecessary loss of life).

In medicine, achieving the prime directive is a multifaceted process. It begins with comprehensive education and training, where physicians and healthcare providers acquire a deep understanding of the human body, diseases, and treatments. This education equips them to make informed decisions that minimize harm to patients.

The practice of medicine should be evidence-based, meaning that treatments and interventions are grounded in scientific research and have been proven safe and effective. Before any treatment is administered, obtaining informed consent from the patient is vital. This involves informing the patient about potential risks, benefits, and alternatives.

Regular reviews and audits of practices and outcomes are important for identifying any potential harm caused to patients and for facilitating continuous improvement in care. Adherence to ethical guidelines, such as respecting patient autonomy, maintaining confidentiality, and promoting patient welfare, is a requirement of the medical profession.

Every intervention carries some risk, so healthcare providers must conduct risk-benefit analyses to ensure the best outcome for the patient. Clear and effective communication between practitioners and patients is crucial, and patients should feel comfortable asking questions and expressing concerns.

As medicine is a rapidly evolving field, continuous learning and professional development are necessary to remain up-to-date on the latest research and treatment options. Patient care often involves a team of professionals, so effective teamwork and clear communication among team members can help prevent errors and harm.

Lastly, each patient is unique, and their values and preferences should be taken into consideration for tailored, individualized care. This approach ensures the best outcomes and minimizes harm.

The maxim "First, do no harm" acts as a key directive in the field of medicine, yet there are instances where its straightforward application may prove difficult. These circumstances should not be viewed as exceptions but rather as intricate situations that necessitate careful and nuanced decisions. For instance, there may be cases where short-term harm is inflicted to attain long-term benefits, such as administering chemotherapy to cancer patients, or undertaking surgeries that inherently carry harmful risks. However, the absence of such interventions could potentially lead to even more detrimental outcomes.

The mindless civilization portrayed in "Return of the Archons" was barely thriving. Spock described the culture as "soulless," without any spirit or spark. Disobeying the prime directive was not only "logical" but necessary to reawaken its creativity. Similar to the medical prime directive, the goal remains to minimize harm as much as possible and to always act in people's best interests.

27

Reflections on "Space Seed," "Paradise Lost," and the Practice of Medicine

The "God Complex" in medicine is mirrored in classic and contemporary literature and cinema.

"Space Seed" is a classic "Star Trek" episode where the crew of the Starship Enterprise encounters a derelict ship, the SS Botany Bay, carrying genetically engineered superhumans in suspended animation from Earth's 20th century. The leader of these superhumans is Khan Noonien Singh—simply known as "Khan"—a charismatic, intelligent, and manipulative figure who once ruled over a significant portion of earth during the 1990s.

Khan attempts to take over the Enterprise but is ultimately defeated and exiled to a remote planet that "is a bit savage [and] somewhat inhospitable," according to Mr. Spock. Captain Kirk turns to Khan and asks, "Can you tame a world?" Khan's rejoinder is, "Have you ever read Milton, Captain?" Scotty admits to not being "up" on Milton, so Kirk explains that Khan's question is in reference to John Milton's epic poem "Paradise Lost," namely, the statement Lucifer made when he fell into the pit: "It is better to rule in hell than serve in heaven."

Spock tells Kirk that "It would be interesting...to return to that world in a hundred years and to learn what crop has sprung from the seed you planted today," meaning to return to the planet that Khan was exiled to in order to see if he was able to tame it. "Yes, Mister Spock, it would indeed," marvels Kirk. The show's ending perfectly sets the stage for the later film "Star Trek II: The Wrath of Khan," where Khan is famously played (again) by Ricardo Montalbán.

"Paradise Lost" tells the biblical story of the fall of mankind, exploring the temptation of Adam and Eve by the fallen angel Satan and their subsequent expulsion from the Garden of Eden. It is renowned for its complex characters and exploration of themes as seen in "Space Seed," such as power, temptation, and evil. "Paradise Lost" is particularly noted for its sympathetic portrayal of Satan, often considered a tragic figure doomed by his pride.

Certain features of "Paradise Lost" and "Space Seed" can be applied to the practice of medicine in thematic and philosophical ways. One of the main themes in both is the concept of free will and responsibility. In "Paradise Lost," the exercise of free will by Adam and Eve leads to the fall of mankind. Similarly, in medicine, patients have the autonomy to make decisions about their treatment, highlighting the significance and repercussions of personal choices.

Another connection is the role of knowledge. In the poem, the forbidden fruit represents knowledge that results in the loss of innocence for Adam and Eve. In the medical field, knowledge can serve as both a relief and a source of fear and anxiety, such as when a diagnosis is made.

Furthermore, "Paradise Lost" ends with the promise of redemption through Jesus Christ, which can be likened to the role of physicians in promoting healing and recovery. Just as redemption provides hope for mankind in the poem, medical treatments offer hope to patients battling illnesses.

The complexity of good and evil is also a central theme in both. Milton's sympathetic portrayal of Satan reflects how medical ethics often deal with complex moral dilemmas where the line between right and wrong is blurred.

Finally, the shared experience of suffering in "Paradise Lost" and in patient experiences underlines the importance of compassion in the practice of medicine. Thus, "Paradise Lost" provides a rich array of themes that resonate deeply with the medical field.

It is obvious from reading the poem why some physicians develop a "God complex." The term "God complex" is often used to describe individuals, including some physicians, who behave as if they are infallible or possess superior knowledge or abilities. This can lead to a lack of consideration for the opinions or feelings of others, including patients.

In "Paradise Lost," the character of Satan could potentially be seen as having a "God complex." He is portrayed as a proud, ambitious figure who seeks to challenge God's authority, and who believes he is right in doing so. This could be related to some physicians who, due to their specialized knowledge and the life-and-death nature of their work, may develop an inflated sense of their own abilities and importance.

Additionally, the poem's exploration of knowledge and its consequences are particularly relevant to medical practice. Just as the pursuit of forbidden knowledge leads to the fall of mankind. physicians have access to vast amounts of medical knowledge and often make critical decisions based on this knowledge. This responsibility can sometimes lead to an inflated sense of self-importance, similar to a "God complex."

Returning to "Space Seed," one can easily see how Khan, a genetically enhanced superhuman, would possess a god-like belief in his own superiority. Khan's desire for power and control echo Satan's ambition in "Paradise Lost." Both characters challenge the existing order, resulting in dire consequences. Similarly, physicians who disregard their patients' autonomy and make decisions without their input can cause harm, highlighting the importance of recognizing the limits of one's abilities and knowledge.

Furthermore, Khan's enhanced knowledge and abilities can be seen as a double-edged sword, much like the forbidden fruit in "Paradise Lost" and the medical knowledge physicians possess. While this knowledge can be beneficial, it can also lead to overconfidence and potentially harmful decisions.

Finally, the theme of compassion is evident in "Space Seed," particularly in the character of Lt. Marla McGivers (played by Madlyn Rhue). McGivers is the USS Enterprise historian who sympathizes with Khan despite his actions and is exiled with him. This mirrors the compassion that is crucial in the practice of medicine, as well as Adam and Eve's experience of suffering in "Paradise Lost."

In conclusion, "Space Seed" shares several themes with "Paradise Lost," and both raise issues applicable to the practice of medicine, including the potential pitfalls of a "God complex," the double-edged sword of knowledge, and the importance of compassion. However, it is important to note that such a complex is not representative of most physicians. Only a narcissist like Khan could refer to McGivers as a "superior woman" and quip, "I will take her." If he were a physician, he would no doubt be reported for misconduct.

28

What Makes Healthcare Executives Exceptional?

The best healthcare executives distinguish themselves through leadership, communication, and emotional intelligence.

Considering what I wrote in essay 5 and what lies ahead in essay 45, you'll notice that I do not hold healthcare executives in especially high regard. But of course, there are exceptions.

One of the best I worked under came at the tail end of my career. He was a kind and compassionate man, highly principled and devoted to his faith and family. He sent a company-wide email upon his resignation from the organization. I've de-identified the letter yet preserved its essence. Here is his communication:

"Dear Team,

I wanted to let you know of information I shared with our Board last night.

After 24 years of work in the public system and having had the privilege to serve as the CEO of our company since 2012, I will be retiring from the position in a few months. I leave with a lot of personal excitement about what lies ahead for me and my wife and with professional confidence that great things are ahead for our organization.

On a professional level, I am proud of a lot of things as I think back about my last 12 years as CEO. Three things though stand out and will be things I will always cherish. First, I am proud of our mission. We have been committed to truly improving lives and strengthening communities, and that is important and means a lot. Our mission is noble, we have made a difference for many, and we have been true to our purpose. For that, I am proud.

Secondly, I am proud of our team. I have had a front row seat to watch the expertise and professionalism of so many smart and talented people. No matter what the need, what the challenge, or how demanding the moment has been, our incredible and dedicated professionals have excelled. I have been honored and have learned a lot from being surrounded by the incredible individuals that make our organization so special.

Lastly, I am proud of never compromising the integrity with which we have pursued our mission. We have not been perfect, and we have learned through those moments of opportunity, but we have never faltered and never wavered from doing things the right way and with the utmost integrity in our efforts.

The Board of Directors has already begun their process to transition to the next CEO and will be executing their plan during the coming weeks. I applaud the Board for their steadfast commitment to the stability of our company while ensuring that we reach greater success as we look ahead. As they have directed, I will advise them during this process and will ensure a smooth handoff to the successor when they are ready to announce that decision.

Until then, and beyond, we have a lot to do and accomplish and I look forward to us remaining locked arm in arm to ensure that success. Thanks for what you have done, for what you are doing, and for what you will do in the future.

I wish you all the best in all aspects of your lives! Stay committed to your priorities and cherish every moment!

[Name Withheld]"

The CEO did not share his future plans. He is only 60 years old, and he could retire if he chooses, or move on to another position to be closer to his children and grandchildren. I only worked with him for a little over a year. Compared to other healthcare executives, however, he stood out.

Exceptional healthcare executives distinguish themselves through a combination of key qualities. They exhibit strong leadership skills, setting an example for their team and driving them towards shared goals. Their extensive knowledge of the healthcare industry is also critical, as it includes understanding current trends, technologies, and regulatory changes. These executives display strategic thinking, effectively developing and implementing plans that align with the organization's mission and objectives.

Moreover, their communication skills enable them to interact effectively with a range of stakeholders, including physicians, staff, and patients. They also have a firm grasp of the financial aspects of running a healthcare organization, such as budgeting, forecasting, and financial analysis. Their ability to make informed decisions swiftly, even under pressure, is another important trait.

Exceptional healthcare executives are adaptable, capable of leading their organizations through changes and challenges. They prioritize a patient-centric approach, constantly striving to enhance patient care and satisfaction. These executives maintain high ethical standards, ensuring all operations comply with relevant laws and regulations.

Lastly, their emotional intelligence is evident in their empathetic and understanding nature, which helps manage their teams effectively and deal with patients and their families sensitively. They are innovative thinkers, always seeking to improve processes and patient care, and are dedicated to ongoing learning and development.

Whether or not healthcare CEOs are physicians may make little difference in their ability to lead organizations. It is interesting, however, the very best hospitals and health systems, e.g., the Mayo and Cleveland Clinics, are physicians-led. In fact, there are three physician leaders at the helm of the Mayo Clinic, which has major campuses in Arizona, Florida and Minnesota.

Physician-led hospitals outperformed their counterparts in quality of care, cost of care and access to care, according to an NDP Analytics study published in 2022. The findings of course do not prove that doctors make better leaders, though the results are surely consistent with that claim. It may simply be that the separation of clinical and managerial knowledge inside hospitals is associated with worse management.

Doctors were once viewed as ill-prepared for leadership roles because their selection and training led them to become "heroic lone healers." They frequently assumed leadership roles by default, and leadership skills were left largely to chance. But this is changing. The emphasis on patient-centered care and efficiency in the delivery of clinical outcomes means that physicians are now being prepared for leadership and possibly better equipped than nonphysicians to handle the extraordinary challenges of running healthcare organizations.

The balance of quality against cost, and of technology against humanity, are placing ever-increasing value on physicians as leaders, with many recruiters advertising that an MBA degree is a "plus." MD/MBAs do, in fact, command a slightly higher salary than physicians without the MBA. In 2022, there were 92 MD/MBA programs among 151 U.S. medical schools (60.9%).

My friend and colleague Peter Angood, MD, has been CEO of the American Association for Physician Leadership (AAPL) for over a decade. AAPL is considered the "home" for physician leaders and equips physicians with the skills necessary to become effective leaders. Membership in AAPL has grown over the years, reflecting physicians' keen interest in assuming CEO and other leadership positions, especially chief medical officer.

Angood believes that all physicians are leaders at some level. I, too, believe his statement is true. However, it is not unreasonable for physicians to emulate great nonphysician leaders and learn from them as well. The CEO I worked for was a fine example.

29

Dealing with Discouragement: Strategies for Aspiring Medical Students

Overcome the negativity of authority figures in your life.

Do you remember times when your dreams, hopes, and aspirations were crushed by teachers and other authority figures? We've all encountered such times. These experiences shape our character in negative ways and can lead to devastating psychological effects. This kind of negative influence can greatly impact our self-esteem and self-worth, instilling a deep-seated fear of failure. It can cause us to question our abilities and potential, leading to imposter syndrome (psychological pattern in which individuals doubt their accomplishments and have a persistent fear of being exposed as a fraud, despite evidence of their competence and success).

Repeated discouragement may cause us to develop a negative outlook on life, feel hopeless, and lose motivation to pursue our goals. Furthermore, defeating encounters with authority figures can result in an aversion to them, which can affect our future interactions and relationships. The psychological trauma caused by such experiences can hinder personal growth and development, stifling our potential to thrive. It is, therefore, crucial to seek out positive role models who will foster a supportive and encouraging environment to nurture our dreams and aspirations instead of crushing them.

I know first-hand that if a premedical advisor tells you, "You'll never get into medical school," the psychological impacts can be profoundly damaging. Such negative feedback can shatter your self-confidence, potentially giving up on your dream of becoming a doctor.

Worse yet, you might develop anxiety or depression due to the perceived rejection and the seeming impossibility of achieving your goal. This sense of hopelessness can further lead to a decline in academic performance and a lack of motivation to pursue your aspirations. The impact of discouraging words from a trusted advisor can be long-lasting and detrimental, stifling your potential and hindering your personal and professional development.

It is important to note that a premedical advisor's role should be to guide and support you, not discourage you. Constructive feedback can be helpful, but it should be offered in a way that encourages improvement rather than causes demotivation. If you are as determined as I was to pursue a career in medicine, you should seek second opinions, take advantage of resources and support systems, and continue to work hard towards your goal.

"You'll never get into medical school" was a defeatist comment uttered by my premedical advisor in my junior year of college. She made the statement in the context of my grades—a B+ average—and for taking the bare minimum of science courses. She was correct. I was roundly rejected by all medical schools on my first go-around. But I was determined to prove her wrong—and I did!

I did something unorthodox. I called a doctor who had interviewed me at one of the medical schools I had applied to, and I asked for his advice. Not only did he accept my phone call, but he also extended a welcoming invitation to discuss my situation over morning coffee at his home (we lived in the same city). He said he remembered me from the interview and he enjoyed reading my application essay, but my grades and MCAT scores needed to improve. He suggested that during my gap year, I do what was necessary to boost my grade point average and MCAT scores, and if I were successful, he would present me to the admissions committee. His advice worked, and I was offered admission.

I count my lucky stars that an admissions officer would reach out to me and provide clear guidance and genuine hospitality. No other medical school offered me admission on my second try. If it weren't for the kindness of strangers, I probably wouldn't have become a doctor. Of course, I persevered and had the chutzpah to contact him during my gap year and keep him abreast of my progress, but this physician more than met me halfway.

I understand that the journey towards becoming a medical professional can be filled with various challenges, including discouragement from others. It's essential to know that this does not define your potential or ability to succeed in your medical career. Your journey into medicine is unique to you, and your potential is not defined by the negative comments of others. I have several strategies to help you navigate through such situations.

Maintaining a positive mindset is your first line of defense against discouragement. The power of positivity can help you stay focused on your goals and not let negativity hinder your progress. It's also beneficial to seek mentorship from seasoned professionals, teachers, or anyone who can provide valuable guidance and encouragement. They can offer insights and advice that will help you navigate your path to medical school.

If you find that certain areas of your application need improvement, don't hesitate to address them. Whether it's working towards better grades, gaining clinical experience, or refining your personal statement, every improvement counts. Preparing for the MCAT is also critical, as a high score can significantly increase your chances of acceptance.

Remember to broaden your horizons when applying to medical schools. Different schools have different selection criteria, and you might find an institution that values your unique strengths, even if it's overseas. Persistence is key in this journey. Setbacks are inevitable, but it's your resilience and determination that will ultimately determine your success.

Lastly, the importance of self-care cannot be overstated. During this demanding period, taking care of your mental and physical health is vital. It's cliché to say, but regular exercise, a balanced diet, and sufficient rest will help you remain focused and motivated on your journey.

Always remember that many successful medical professionals have faced similar obstacles and discouragement. It's essential not to let the opinions of others deter you from your dreams. You are the only one who can shape your future, whether it be in the medical field or elsewhere.

30

From Resident to Academic Attending: The Challenges Ahead

With appropriate support, this can be a time of growth and learning.

I transitioned to attending status immediately after I completed my residency. One day, I was chief resident. The next day, I was an attending physician—at the same academic center. Transitioning from a resident to an attending physician is both exciting and rewarding. After years of rigorous training, doctors are finally able to practice independently. However, this new role comes with its own set of trials. Many of them are psychological in nature.

The Challenges Ahead

One of the biggest changes is the shift in responsibility. As an attending physician, you are the final decision-maker in patient care. While the autonomy can be liberating, it can also be daunting as the full weight of patient outcomes rests on your shoulders. There is no longer a safety net of a more experienced doctor to double-check decisions or to turn to for immediate advice. This can sometimes lead to "impostor syndrome," where you may doubt your abilities and feel like a fraud, despite your qualifications and training.

Another challenge can be managing time. Balancing the need to guide and teach a team of residents and medical students, while also ensuring high-quality patient care, can be a difficult juggling act.

If you are obligated to do research to fulfill the tripartite mission of your academic medical center, time pressure will become even greater and may overwhelm you.

Don't be fooled into thinking that the workload will decrease because you can rely on the house staff to ease the clinical burden. Recall that the Fat Man in *The House of God* suggests that the best thing a medical student can do for a resident is to not do anything at all. The implication is that medical students, because of their lack of experience, may unintentionally create more work or complications for the residents, hence not saving them time. The same is sometimes true regarding the relationship between residents and attendings.

Furthermore, any time saved by doing less direct patient care may be offset by the administrative demands of patient care that fall to attendings, including paperwork, meetings, and dealing with insurance companies. This can lead to long hours and potential burnout if not managed effectively.

A Fine Balancing Act of Leadership and Responsibility

Navigating the politics and hierarchy of academia can be tricky. Building relationships with nursing staff, administrators, and other physicians is crucial for success as an attending. Ultimately, you want to be known as a "triple A" doctor, one who is Able, Affable, and Available, proud to add "AAA" after your MD or DO degree. The display of a happy façade and genial demeanor does not come naturally for some doctors.

Because I chose to stay at the academic center where I was both a medical student and a resident, my issue was not forging new relationships as much as it was wanting to be viewed as an expert in the eyes of those who had trained me. I did not want to disappoint them or fall short of their expectations. However, after years of being a low man on the totem pole—an attending 8 years in the making—I found it difficult to work my way up.

Nurses and other attendings still tended to relate to me in their default mode (i.e., as if I were still a trainee). I felt pressure to demonstrate my competence and dispel any prior misconceptions about my abilities. In order to be seen in a new light, I had to act with authority and assume the role of an opinion leader.

At the same time, I had to check my ego at the door. Sure, I wanted to wax eloquent with students and residents on rounds and refer them to the latest research articles to justify my treatment recommendations. (And I did that—the residents nicknamed me "Article" Lazarus.) But I also had to demonstrate humility and not lull myself into thinking I knew more about the practice of medicine (psychiatry) than I really did. I had to remind myself I, too, was learning, and that although I was well-versed in the clinical treatment of disease, I was still figuring out how to best manage patients' expectations and those of the people I worked with.

As a newly minted attending, you must take on a leader's role and orchestrate a multidisciplinary team of healthcare professionals. Leadership requires a shift in professional identity and extensive practical experience to adapt to the new role of attending. There is no way to rush the process. Yet, identity formation can take time and may involve introspection and mentorship. Most physicians do not receive regular, structured, professional mentorship or coaching. Leadership is simply expected of attendings from the beginning, like flipping a switch, which is unrealistic. The pairing of a new attending with a senior mentor who provides regular advice and support could be invaluable.

New attendings often have a difficult time seeking clinical consultation. I was reluctant to ask for advice lest it make me appear less competent or knowledgeable. When a new attending asks for help it may be perceived as a weakness, whereas help-seeking behavior initiated by a senior physician, one who has already proven themselves, is often viewed as a sign of strength and camaraderie. You will have to go it alone for some time to earn your stripes before you can join the ranks of the privileged and comfortably eat with them at the faculty dining room.

An Opportunity for Learning and Growth

My transition to the attending role coincided with life changes that are typical at this early stage of career development, such as starting a family, paying off student loans, and studying for specialty boards. All of these events can cause stress. Many doctors take up attending positions in new cities or even new countries, and adjusting to a new location, building a new social network, and navigating a new healthcare system or hospital can be an additional source of anxiety. This is yet another reason to seek a mentor or coach, someone who can help you navigate the complexities of your career.

Overall, the shift from resident to attending physician is a significant milestone that brings about many personal and professional changes. It is rarely seamless and, in fact, often accompanied by worries and self-doubt. Navigating these psychological challenges requires self-awareness, resilience, and support from mentors, colleagues, and loved ones. With appropriate support, this can be a time of growth and learning, both in and out of the hospital.

While the transition from resident to attending can be challenging, with time you are bound to adapt to your new roles and responsibilities, solidifying your position while finding your own style of practicing medicine.

31

The Impact of War Trauma, the Challenge of Objectivity, and the Power of Therapy and Storytelling in Healing

*Storytelling can be an effective medium
for managing war trauma.*

Trauma in the form of war is one of the worst forms of trauma to endure. How do people remain objective about events and the involved nations when they have been directly or indirectly affected by war?

For example, how are Holocaust survivors and their families able to relate unemotionally to present-day German citizens? How do the descendants of the more than 2,000 allied civilians who were imprisoned in the infamous Japanese-controlled Weihsien (China) Internment Camp look upon today's Japanese nationals dispassionately? How can one criticize Israel's rampage of Gaza without being labeled antisemitic or feeling the need to run amok on college campuses and threaten Jewish students?

War trauma, with its profound psychological distress, can significantly impact an individual's perception of events and countries involved in the conflict. This trauma can be experienced directly through personal exposure to war or indirectly through the suffering of loved ones. The after-effects often persist long after the conflict has ended, leading to a range of mental health issues including posttraumatic stress disorder (PTSD) and depression.

Maintaining objectivity in the wake of such trauma is undoubtedly challenging. However, several strategies can assist individuals in this process. Psychoeducation plays a crucial role in helping individuals understand the nature of trauma and its impact on mental health. This understanding can lay the groundwork for a more objective analysis of events and nations.

Professional therapeutic interventions such as cognitive (or dialectical) behavioral therapy (C/DBT) and eye movement desensitization and reprocessing (EMDR) can be instrumental in dealing with trauma. These techniques can help individuals restructure their thoughts and emotions, allowing them to view events from a more objective standpoint.

Practices like mindfulness and meditation can also be beneficial. By helping individuals stay grounded in the present moment, these practices can minimize the influence of past trauma on current perceptions.

A strong support system, encompassing friends, family, or support groups, can provide varying perspectives and a safe space for discussion. This facilitation can encourage the development of a more objective viewpoint.

Gaining education and exposure to different cultures, histories, and perspectives can foster understanding and empathy. This appears to be critically absent from the war between Israel and Hamas, fueling tensions and preventing individuals from forming a more balanced view of the conflict.

In addition to the therapeutic interventions and strategies already mentioned, medication may play a crucial role in managing the symptoms of trauma and promoting objectivity. Pharmacotherapy can be beneficial in managing the symptoms of both PTSD and depression, as well as various anxiety disorders that may accompany trauma.

For instance, selective serotonin reuptake inhibitors (SSRIs) and serotonin and norepinephrine reuptake inhibitors (SNRIs) are often used to treat these conditions. These medications can help regulate mood, reduce anxiety, and improve overall well-being, thus providing a more stable emotional platform from which to view events objectively.

Antipsychotic medications may also be used in some cases, particularly when individuals are experiencing severe symptoms such as hallucinations or delusions. Antipsychotics are also used to augment the potential of antidepressants, especially in individuals whose depression proves difficult to treat. Modern, "second-generation" antipsychotic drugs can help to stabilize the individual's mental state and improve their ability to perceive reality accurately.

It is important to note, however, that the use of medication should always be considered as part of a comprehensive treatment plan that includes the psychotherapeutic modalities discussed above. Furthermore, the decision to use medication should be made collaboratively between the physician and the patient, taking into account the individual's specific symptoms, overall health status, and personal preferences. It is also vital to remember that healing from trauma is a gradual and individual process. Each person's circumstances should be approached with patience, empathy, and respect for the individual's personal journey.

Because recovery from trauma is unique to the individual, storytelling has emerged as an effective therapeutic tool in helping individuals process and cope with the psychological distress. It provides a safe and structured platform for expressing emotions related to traumatic experiences. This form of expression can offer relief and reduce symptoms of distress. The "story shepherds" of war-torn Northern Ireland can attest to the healing power of storytelling.

Storytelling has also been instrumental for many Holocaust survivors. The act of sharing their experiences—"Shoah testimony"—has served multiple purposes, both for the survivors themselves and for society at large. Storytelling has been a way for survivors to reclaim their identities, to sustain their resilience and strength, and to come to terms with the unimaginable events they lived through.

Narration provides a sense of control and self-affirmation. By narrating their experiences, Holocaust survivors have been able to contextualize their suffering and find some form of closure. Moreover, the stories serve as a powerful warning against the dangers of hatred, prejudice, and indifference. They remind us of our responsibility to uphold human rights and prevent such atrocities from happening again.

Storytelling encourages cognitive processing. As individuals recount their experiences, they can gain a better understanding of their trauma, helping them to reframe their experiences, challenge negative beliefs, and develop a more balanced perspective. Storytelling also fosters a sense of connection and empathy among those who have experienced similar traumas. This shared experience can reduce feelings of isolation and provide a supportive community. In addition, the act of telling one's story can be empowering. It helps preserve personal and collective memories of traumatic events, whereas repressing them may hinder the healing process.

The integration of storytelling into therapeutic interventions can take various forms (refer to essay 7), such as narrative therapy, writing exercises, or group therapy sessions. Digital media like video or audio recordings can also facilitate storytelling, providing a platform for wider sharing and advocacy. Although storytelling is a powerful tool in managing war trauma, it should be facilitated with sensitivity, respecting each individual's readiness to share and their unique narrative.

32

Unmasking the "Lost" Mental Health Generation

Many adults have been retrospectively diagnosed with autism, ADHD, and bipolar disorder.

The term "Lost Generation" was initially used to describe the generation that came of age during World War I, popularized by Ernest Hemingway. It referenced the disillusionment experienced by many, especially intellectuals and creatives, who lived through the war and its aftermath.

Several decades later, the term was applied to another group. The "Woodstock Generation" typically refers to the Baby Boomers, specifically those who were young adults in the 1960s and 1970s during the time of the famous Woodstock Music Festival in 1969. They are sometimes referred to as the "Lost Generation" in a cultural or societal context, as they challenged many conventional norms and values during a time of significant societal upheaval.

In the context of mental health, the term "Lost Generation" was coined in a seminal 2015 paper published in *The Lancet Psychiatry* to refer to adults with autism spectrum disorder (ASD) who were not diagnosed as children. More recently the phrase has been broadened to include adults who have been retrospectively diagnosed with other developmental and mental health disorders, such as attention deficit/hyperactivity disorder (ADHD) and bipolar disorder.

The Lost Generation in Mental Health

The "lost" mental health generation primarily comprises individuals who were children before the late 20th century, a period when awareness and understanding of ASD, ADHD, and bipolar disorder were significantly less than today and diagnostic criteria were not precise—or they were non-existent (e.g., the term "minimal brain dysfunction" was commonly substituted for ADHD). During this time, these conditions were often misdiagnosed as behavioral issues or personality traits, leading to inappropriate treatment or no treatment at all during their formative years.

Notably, the prevalence of autism in children is just under 3%, but neurodivergent traits in the general population (including autism, OCD, ADHD, dyslexia, and others) can be found in as many as 15-20%.

Autistic adults may go unrecognized or be diagnosed late in life, particularly physicians. In one study, 10% of patients at an institution had autism but went unidentified; they never received a proper diagnosis. In fact, autistic adults are about 30 times less likely than children to be diagnosed. The word "autism" didn't appear in the Diagnostic and Statistical Manual of Mental Disorders until 1980.

The Impact of No or Delayed Diagnosis

Individuals who have grown up without a proper diagnosis often struggle with symptoms that were misunderstood or overlooked during their childhood years. This late diagnosis can have significant implications for their social, professional, and personal lives. They might have struggled with school, work, relationships, and self-esteem due to unrecognized symptoms. Not understanding why they felt or acted differently from their peers could have led to feelings of isolation, alienation, and resentment.

Furthermore, these individuals may have missed out on early interventions and treatments that could have improved their quality of life. This could include behavioral therapies, medication, and educational accommodations that are typically more effective when started early in life.

It is a well-documented fact that many adults with conditions like ASD, ADHD, and bipolar disorder have developed various coping mechanisms and strategies to hide their symptoms. This phenomenon, often referred to as "camouflaging" or "masking," involves individuals consciously or subconsciously managing their behavior to fit in with societal norms or expectations.

Masking behavior is particularly common among adults with ASD, including forcing eye contact during conversations, learning to script responses in social situations, or suppressing stimming (self-stimulatory behaviors like hand flapping or rocking). Some autistic individuals may also develop elaborate strategies to avoid situations that could reveal their autism, such as eschewing spontaneous social events where they cannot predict the behavior expected of them.

These behaviors can make it challenging for others, including medical professionals, to recognize signs of autism in adults, contributing to late or missed diagnoses. Also, while masking can help autistic individuals navigate social situations, it often comes at a significant psychological cost. The constant effort to appear neurotypical can be mentally and emotionally exhausting, leading to high levels of stress, anxiety, and even burnout, which can exacerbate mental health issues and contribute to the high rates of depression and anxiety disorders seen in adults with ASD.

In the case of ADHD, adults may develop strategies to manage their symptoms such as using calendars, alarms, and other tools to stay organized. They might also choose careers or lifestyles that accommodate their need for high levels of activity.

For those with bipolar disorder, some individuals may learn to recognize their mood swings and take steps to mitigate their impact.

Story Treasures

They might isolate themselves during manic or depressive episodes, or they may overcompensate during their more stable periods to maintain their relationships and responsibilities.

While masking and coping mechanisms can make individuals with all three disorders appear neurotypical, they do not eliminate the underlying condition. This highlights the importance of early diagnosis and intervention, so individuals can receive the support they need without having to resort to constant camouflaging. It also underscores the need for societal acceptance and understanding of neurodiversity, which would reduce the pressure on autistic individuals to camouflage their natural behaviors.

Implications for Health Professionals

The rise in adult diagnoses of ASD, ADHD, and bipolar disorder has significant implications for mental health professionals. It underscores the need for improved training and awareness of these conditions in adults, as well as the development of appropriate diagnostic tools and treatment strategies for this population.

Moreover, it highlights the importance of considering these diagnoses when working with adults who present with complex mental health issues, particularly those with a history of unsuccessful treatments.

The "lost" generation of adults retrospectively diagnosed with ASD, ADHD, and bipolar disorder serves as an important reminder of the progress we've made in mental health awareness and diagnosis. However, it also emphasizes the need for continued efforts in improving early detection, intervention, and support for individuals with these conditions, regardless of their age.

33

Generation Z and Implications for Medical Education

Educators must adopt best practices to prepare for a new generation of doctors.

Generation Z—individuals born between 1997 and 2012—makes up one-fifth of the U.S. population. "Gen Z" is the most diverse generation in history in terms of race, gender, and sexual orientation. Environmental, social, and governance practices with a focus on sustainability and diversity, equity, and inclusion (DEI) initiatives are critically important to this generation, colloquially known as "Zoomers." Many do not remember a time before smartphones and social media; hence, Gen Zers have also been dubbed the iGeneration. Gen Z individuals undoubtedly bring unique challenges and opportunities to the domain of education and medical education in particular.

As digital natives, Gen Z students have an inherent understanding of technology, using it for learning, information gathering, and communication from a young age. This familiarity with technology suggests that traditional lecture-based teaching may not be as effective. Instead, a shift towards more interactive, technology-driven educational methods, such as online platforms, virtual simulations, and digital anatomy tools, may be required.

Indeed, a 2024 poll conducted by Zing Coach found that 56% of Gen Z respondents use TikTok for wellness, diet and fitness advice and that a large share of them use the platform as their main form of health advice. Among those surveyed—1,000 people aged 18 to 27—34% said they use TikTok to get most of their health advice, making it more than twice as popular as the other options listed.

Research also shows that Generation Z's attention span is considerably shorter than that of their predecessors—even compared to goldfish—possibly due to their regular interaction with quick, concise information through social media and other digital platforms. These findings imply that medical education may need to adopt more engaging, brief, and interactive teaching methods.

Generation Z tends to be visual learners, preferring images, videos, and infographics over traditional text-heavy materials. Medical educators should consider incorporating visual aids and multimedia resources to enhance learning retention and comprehension.

Authenticity and transparency in all matters, especially education, are highly valued by Gen Zers. They seek real-world relevance in their learning experiences. Medical educators should emphasize the practical application of knowledge, provide opportunities for clinical exposure and hands-on skills training, and foster open communication and collaboration between students and faculty.

Because Generation Z is the most diverse generation yet, a strong emphasis on inclusivity and social justice is welcomed in the teaching curriculum. Medical education should reflect this diversity and promote cultural competence, empathy, and awareness of social determinants of health to prepare future health care professionals to serve diverse patient populations effectively.

Generation Z is entrepreneurial and values creativity, innovation, and autonomy. Medical education can encourage entrepreneurial thinking by integrating courses on health care innovation, entrepreneurship, and leadership skills development, empowering students to drive positive change in health care delivery and research. Medical schools should strive to build partnerships with humanities and business departments in their parent universities and incorporate selective courses to complement basic science classes.

Generation Z students place a high value on personalization and expect their educational experiences to be tailored to their individual interests and career aspirations. This desire for customization further challenges the traditional structure and standardization of medical education. Therefore, medical schools might need to consider more flexible curricula and individualized learning pathways. The importance of extracurricular and community-building activities cannot be understated.

Another notable characteristic of Generation Z is their higher levels of stress and anxiety compared to previous generations. Factors such as academic pressure, social media use, and contemporary global uncertainties could contribute to these mental health issues. Indeed, the unsettling war in the Middle East discussed in essay 31 is perhaps a harbinger of the way future ethnic conflicts will play out and is all the more reason to make mental health resources available to students.

The stark reality, however, is that Generation Z has already faced stressors such as 9/11, school shootings, climate change, and a global pandemic. Thus, they are more open about mental health issues and seek support to address mental well-being. Medical education should prioritize the promotion of student wellness, resilience, and self-care practices, while also providing education on mental health assessment, intervention, and de-stigmatization.

Growing up in a connected world means Generation Z has taken on a global perspective and special interest in global health issues. Medical education should, therefore, incorporate global health perspectives, cultural competency training, and opportunities for international experiences to prepare students for the realities of practicing medicine in an interconnected world. Residency programs should prepare doctors for locum tenens assignments to fill staffing gaps in underserved and war-torn areas.

As important as politics is to today's current events, the debates and events that will ultimately shape Generation Z are likely yet to be known. What does seem clear, however, is that significant educational adjustments are required to meet the unique challenges of this generation as they consider a career in medicine. These can also be seen as opportunities for innovation and progress.

In summary, adapting medical education to meet the needs and preferences of Generation Z requires innovative approaches that leverage technology, active learning strategies, visual content, authenticity, diversity, and inclusion. By recognizing and responding to the learning preferences and needs of Generation Z, medical schools can enhance their educational curricula and better equip future physicians for the evolving health care landscape.

34

Conscious and Unconscious Aspects of Storytelling

Juxtaposing the writings of Federico García Lorca and Carl Jung.

The renowned Spanish poet and playwright Federico García Lorca wrote, "The poem, the song, the picture, is only water drawn from the well of the people, and it should be given back to them in a cup of beauty so that they may drink—and in drinking understand themselves." It suggests that every story, whether it is in the form of a narrative, a poem, a song, or a picture, is derived from the collective consciousness of the people. The power of storytelling in medicine is its ability to draw from the collective, transform it into something beautiful, and then use it to enlighten and heal the people it drew from, to see their thoughts, feelings, and experiences reflected back at them in a new and healthier light.

The notion that stories can be born from the collective experiences, emotions, and aspirations of people calls forth another quote by the famous psychiatrist Carl Jung. Jung wrote, "There is no coming to consciousness without pain. People will do anything, no matter how absurd, in order to avoid facing their own soul. One does not become enlightened by imagining figures of light, but by making the darkness conscious."

This quote suggests that true consciousness and self-realization often emerge from confronting the darker aspects of ourselves, rather than seeking solace in illusions or superficial enlightenment. Growth and understanding require facing the discomfort and pain that accompany self-reflection. Avoiding this process leads people to engage in various distractions or illusions to evade confronting their inner truths. True enlightenment arises from embracing the shadows within us and integrating them into our consciousness. By acknowledging and understanding our darkness, we can truly illuminate our path towards personal growth and enlightenment.

Storytelling often serves as a medium through which individuals explore and confront the complexities of the human condition, including the darker aspects of the psyche. Just as Jung's quote emphasizes the importance of facing one's own soul and making the darkness conscious, storytelling frequently involves characters grappling with their inner conflicts, fears, and vulnerabilities.

In literature, films, and other forms of storytelling, protagonists often undergo journeys of self-discovery and transformation that parallel the process of coming to consciousness described in the quote. They confront their own shadows, face adversity, and ultimately achieve growth and enlightenment through their experiences.

Moreover, stories have the power to evoke empathy and understanding in audiences by presenting nuanced portrayals of characters struggling with their inner demons. Through engaging with these narratives, audiences may also be prompted to reflect on their own lives and confront aspects of themselves they may have avoided.

Storytelling and Jung's concept of the collective unconscious are deeply intertwined. Jung proposed that the collective unconscious is a reservoir of shared, universal symbols, archetypes, and patterns of thought that are inherent to all humans, regardless of culture or upbringing. These archetypes manifest in myths, legends, folklore, and, by extension, in storytelling.

Many of the themes, characters, and motifs found in stories resonate with the archetypes of the collective unconscious. For example, the hero's journey archetype, which entails a protagonist leaving the ordinary world, facing challenges, and returning transformed, is prevalent in numerous myths and narratives across cultures. Similarly, archetypal figures such as the wise old mentor, the trickster, and the shadow are common in storytelling worldwide.

Through storytelling, individuals tap into the collective unconscious, both as creators and as audiences. Storytellers draw upon archetypal elements to craft narratives that resonate with universal human experiences and emotions. Audiences, in turn, connect with these stories on a deep, subconscious level, recognizing and responding to the archetypal patterns present within them.

Moreover, storytelling serves as a means of collective expression and exploration of the collective unconscious. By sharing and engaging with stories, communities and cultures reinforce their shared values, beliefs, and symbols, thereby perpetuating and enriching the collective unconscious.

Through stories, individuals and societies explore, express, and interact with the archetypal patterns deeply ingrained in the human psyche. In storytelling, we bring to light the shared fears, hopes, and experiences that are not only conscious but also reside in our collective unconscious, contributing to universal aspects of human experience that connect us all.

In essence, storytelling provides a mirror through which individuals can explore the depths of their own souls, confront their darkness, and ultimately strive towards greater self-awareness and enlightenment, echoing the themes articulated in both Lorca's and Jung's writings.

35

Every Picture Paints a Story—and Every Story Paints a Picture

The "art" of medical storytelling involves visualizing its narrative components.

Rod Stewart's smash hit song "Every Picture Tells a Story," and his 1971 breakthrough album by the same name, ranks 172 on *Rolling Stone*'s 2003 list of the 500 greatest albums of all time. In the May 1995 issue of *Mojo*, Stewart said of the song: "I can remember the build-up. You know what the song's about—your early teenage life when you're leaving home and you're exploring the world for yourself." The song's title doesn't appear in the lyrics until the end, where it is repeated 24 times! ("Every picture tells a story, don't it?").

The ancient adage, "Every picture paints a story," is a testament to the power of visual imagery in conveying narratives, emotions, and ideas. This phrase encapsulates the ability of images to tell tales without using a single word, to transport viewers to different realities, and to evoke a myriad of emotions. However, the communicative power of stories should not be underestimated either. In fact, stories can paint pictures just as vividly, if not more so, than images. This is particularly true in the field of medicine, where the art of storytelling becomes an essential tool for understanding, diagnosing, and treating patients.

Stories, by their very nature, are evocative. They are filled with characters, settings, conflicts, and resolutions that stimulate the human imagination. Every narrative detail, from the grandest plot developments to the smallest character quirks, contributes to the construction of a mental image. This is how stories paint pictures. They provide the raw materials—the words, phrases, and sentences—from which readers craft their own unique visual interpretations. Every reader becomes an artist, using their imagination as a canvas and the story as their paint.

In the realm of medicine, storytelling takes on a new level of importance. Medical practitioners rely heavily on patient narratives to gain a comprehensive understanding of their patients' health conditions. These narratives, or medical histories, are essentially stories that patients tell about their bodies and way of thinking. They paint a picture of the patient's health, lifestyle, and symptoms that can help the physician make an accurate diagnosis.

These stories can be incredibly detailed, providing a chronological account of the patient's health. They can describe the onset of symptoms, their progression, and any treatments that have been tried. These narratives can also include information about the patient's lifestyle, such as diet, exercise, and stress levels, which can all play a role in their health. By listening to these stories, physicians can visualize the patient's health journey, making connections between symptoms and potential causes and forming an overall picture of the patient's health.

Moreover, storytelling in medicine extends beyond patient narratives. Case reports, clinical studies, and medical literature are all forms of storytelling that paint pictures of diseases, therapies, and medical phenomena. These narratives provide a structured way for medical professionals to share knowledge, learn from each other's experiences, and build on the collective understanding of medicine.

Painting stories play a crucial role in patient education. Medical professionals often use narratives to explain complex medical conditions and procedures to patients. These stories help to demystify medicine, making it more accessible and understandable to patients. By painting a clear picture of what to expect, stories can alleviate patients' fears, encourage them to take an active role in their health and foster a stronger patient-doctor relationship.

The illustrations that accompany my online narratives and embellish the front covers of my books remind me that stories are powerful tools that can paint vivid pictures in the minds of their audience. Just as every picture paints a story, every story paints a picture—a picture that can illuminate the intricacies of human health, guide medical decision-making, and ultimately improve patient outcomes. Some of the most iconic images in the history of medicine are emblematic of narratives that are deeply intertwined with the evolution of the field.

Thomas Eakins' 1875 painting, "The Gross Clinic," for instance, presents a scene from an operating room at Thomas Jefferson Medical College where Dr. Samuel D. Gross, a prominent American surgeon, performs surgery before medical students. This visual narrative underscores the role of hands-on experience (literally) and observation in medical training and the advent of surgical procedures in disease treatment during the late 19th century. Initially rejected for showing at the 1876 Centennial Exhibition in Philadelphia, "The Gross Clinic" is now recognized as one of the greatest American medical paintings for its uncompromised realism.

In a similar vein, Rembrandt's "The Anatomy Lesson of Dr. Nicolaes Tulp" portrays physicians observing an anatomy lesson, in this case, Tulp explaining the musculature of the arm. This iconic 1632 painting, regarded as one of Rembrandt's early masterpieces, emphasizes the significance of anatomical studies in understanding the human body and the importance of continuous learning in medicine.

"The Lady with the Lamp," painted by Henrietta Rae in 1891, beautifully encapsulates Florence Nightingale's commitment to improving health care conditions and her revolutionary role in the field of nursing. The painting depicts Florence Nightingale during her time in the Crimean War, holding a lamp while checking on wounded soldiers. The lamp she carries is the most significant element of the painting. It not only provides a source of light in the literal darkness, but it also serves as a metaphorical beacon of hope and comfort for the wounded and sick.

Moving from paintings to photographs, "Photograph 51," taken by Rosalind Franklin in 1952, reveals the double-helix structure of DNA. This confirms Watson's and Crick's earlier hypothesis of the double-stranded nature of DNA and enables them to build the first correct model a year later. Franklin's X-ray diffraction image is a prequel to the story of the building blocks of life, leading to a deeper understanding of genetic diseases and paving the way for revolutionary treatments, including biologic drugs and gene therapy.

Wilhelm Conrad Röntgen's first X-ray photograph, taken in 1895, showed the bones of his wife's hand and marked a new era in diagnostic medicine, enabling physicians to look inside the human body non-invasively. This image narrates a story of medical innovation and its transformative potential in patient care, as Röntgen's scientific advancement would ultimately benefit a variety of medical fields.

Lastly, the "Blue Marble" photograph, taken by the Apollo 17 crew on December 7, 1972, from a distance of around 18,300 miles from Earth's surface, tells a story of global health and medicine. By showing our planet in its entirety, it advocates for environmental protection and underscores the interconnectedness of health across nations and the need for global cooperation in addressing health issues. This image has been used to promote global health initiatives and raise awareness about environmental health issues.

Each of these images, in its unique way, narrates the progress of medicine, highlighting key breakthroughs, practices, and perspectives that have shaped the field. They serve as visual reminders of the power of medical innovation and the continuous pursuit of knowledge in improving human health. Paintings remind us that the "art" of medical storytelling involves visualizing its narrative components.

36

Euthanizing Our Pets Teaches Us About Progressive End-of-Life Care

While euthanizing a pet is a deeply painful experience,
it also offers valuable lessons about death and dying.

Euthanizing pets is a challenging experience that many pet owners face at some point. It is a deeply emotional and heartbreaking decision, but it can also provide important lessons about death and dying for humans.

Euthanizing a pet can help us confront and understand the inevitability of death. It teaches us that death is a part of life and that no living being is immune to it. It helps us acknowledge that death is an unavoidable part of the natural cycle of life.

Deciding to euthanize a pet often comes from a place of deep compassion and empathy. It teaches us about the importance of relieving suffering and prioritizing the welfare of our loved ones, even when it involves making difficult decisions.

Euthanizing a pet can be a profound grief experience. It can help us understand the process of mourning and the importance of allowing ourselves the time and space to grieve. It teaches us that it is okay to feel sad and that it's important to express our feelings.

One of the hardest lessons euthanizing a pet teaches us is about acceptance and letting go. It forces us to confront our fear of loss and to accept that we cannot control everything. It teaches us the value of life and cherishing the moments we have with our loved ones as well as the importance of letting go when it is time.

Over the years our family has been a home to more than a dozen pets—cats and dogs—cherished and loved beyond description. None of them died in their sleep due to natural causes. All were euthanized when it became clear their quality of life was rapidly deteriorating and they were failing to thrive. Sometimes there was an obvious underlying condition such as cancer, but mostly the cause was unknown.

"Sully" was our beloved 14-year-old Bernese Mountain dog mix, small for the breed and lacking the characteristic white stripe running up his snout plunging deep into his forehead (Figure). Sully's namesake was the *Monsters, Inc.* character known for his gentle and compassionate nature. My daughter named him "Sully" unaware that Chesley "Sully" Sullenberger was the pilot who landed his disabled airliner on the Hudson River, although our "Sully" was also deemed a miracle, rescued from a puppy mill.

When Sully began to deteriorate—his personality vacated by dementia and subsequently losing control of his hind legs and bowels—we decided not to let nature take its course. When it became time to euthanize him, I remarked to the veterinarian, "I just wish he would die in his sleep."

"Hardly," she replied. "They rarely go that way." She explained that most dogs and cats will have many days of challenging stages of deterioration and pain before they finally pass. "Natural death is neither peaceful nor gentle," she added.

"The same is true for humans," I murmured.

Losing such a big part of your family is never easy. The decision to euthanize a pet is dreaded and difficult, especially if family members are not all in agreement. My wife, for example, has witnessed her mother and grandmother battle prolonged Alzheimer's disease. She makes life and death decisions quicker than me. We are different because my medical education taught me to prolong life. There was much less emphasis on quality of life when I trained in the 1970s and 1980s than there is today.

Regardless, our discussions about euthanasia always involved our children. We continue to include them now as grown adults. They, in turn, include us with their own families when facing the same agonizing decisions. A typical conversation about euthanizing our pets invariably branches into several areas as we strive to reach a unified decision. The process is somewhat analogous to a jury deliberation.

Comparing Euthanasia in Pets versus Humans

First, we compare and contrast euthanasia in pets and humans. We recognize that the emotional and ethical aspects of euthanasia are complex, regardless of whether the subject is a pet or a human. Both situations involve making difficult decisions about ending a life to alleviate suffering or progressive mental or physical deterioration. However, there are significant differences in how society and the medical field approach these situations.

In many parts of the world, euthanasia or assisted suicide for humans is illegal, while euthanasia for pets is not only legal but often seen as a humane choice when the pet is suffering. The ethical considerations surrounding human euthanasia are more complex due to the higher consciousness of humans, their ability to express their wishes, and societal and religious views about the sanctity of human life.

The emotional burden in both cases is immense. However, the grief experienced by a pet owner may be different from the grief experienced by a family member or loved one of a human patient. In both cases, the individual must grapple with feelings of loss, guilt, and bereavement. However, the decision-making process for human euthanasia can be further complicated by the patient's wishes, family dynamics, and legal considerations.

In veterinary medicine, the decision to euthanize is usually made by the pet owner, often guided by the advice of the veterinarian. In contrast, the decision to end a human life involves the patient (where possible), family members, physicians, ethicists, and sometimes legal professionals. The patient's wishes, as expressed in living wills or through healthcare proxies, play a significant role in human euthanasia.

In both human and veterinary medicine, the decision for euthanasia is often considered when the patient's quality of life is poor, and there's little to no hope for improvement. However, the assessment of "quality of life" can be more complex in humans due to their cognitive abilities, emotional states, and personal beliefs.

Euthanasia as a Taboo Subject

Second, our family feels comfortable freely discussing the topic of euthanasia while recognizing that for many the practice of intentionally ending a life to relieve pain and suffering is often considered taboo, particularly when it comes to humans.

In many cultures and religions, life is considered sacred, and ending it, even to alleviate suffering, is seen as morally wrong. These beliefs often stem from the idea that only a higher power has the right to determine when a life should end. While it is generally accepted that humans have a right to a dignified death, the question of who gets to decide when a life is no longer worth living is a contentious one.

For many, the ethical dilemma lies in the potential for misuse or abuse of euthanasia. There are concerns that legalizing euthanasia could lead to situations where it is used inappropriately, such as in cases of severe disability, old age, or even economic burden. Clear guidelines and strict regulations are necessary to ensure that the process is not misused or exploited, particularly in cases involving vulnerable populations like the elderly.

The topic of euthanasia is less taboo when it comes to pets, primarily because animals are not considered to have the same rights or consciousness as humans. The decision to euthanize a pet is often seen as a compassionate act to end an animal's suffering. However, it is important to note that this decision can still be emotionally devastating for pet owners and veterinary professionals.

While the taboo surrounding euthanasia is gradually easing—some estimates indicate 50% of all Americans will live where medical aid in dying is authorized and accessible by 2028—euthanasia remains a sensitive subject that requires careful handling and open, respectful dialogue, which is what our family has always valued during these stressful and emotional times.

The Outcomes of Euthanasia

Third, our family discussions consider the potential outcomes of approaching euthanasia in humans as we do in pets. Applying the same principles of pet euthanasia to humans could potentially ease suffering for those with terminal or debilitating illnesses. It might address inequities in end-of-life healthcare, expand end-of-life healthcare options, and transform the emergency room experience for dying patients. Euthanasia might also provide a sense of control to individuals over their life and death, respecting their autonomy and right to a dignified death.

For loved ones and medical professionals, this approach could alleviate the emotional distress associated with watching a person suffer without the ability to provide relief. However, it might also bring about feelings of guilt or conflict, similar to what pet owners experience when deciding to euthanize their pets. Therefore, emotional support at this time is a prerequisite.

A shift in approach would integrate the option of medical aid in dying into standard practice for patient-directed end-of-life care by expanding outreach, education and technical support for clinicians, medical societies, and residency training programs. This would require significant legal changes, including the legalization and regulation of euthanasia or assisted suicide. Societal changes in how we view life, death, and the right to die would be necessary in order to advocate for a more progressive agenda.

Conclusion

Given that euthanasia is illegal in the majority of the United States, our family discussions have been mostly academic. However, we firmly believe that if we approach human euthanasia as we do with pets, it could potentially change perspectives on end-of-life decisions. The scales are gradually tipping in favor of death with dignity, and I have become less of a holdout over time.

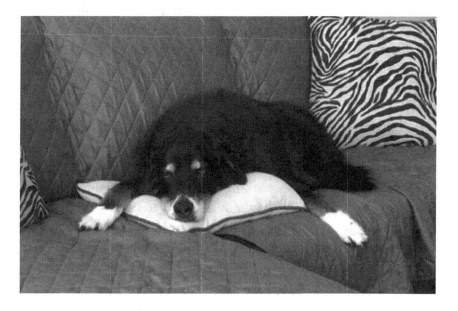

"Sully" (R.I.P.)

37

The Fine Line Between Collecting and Hoarding

The key difference between them is the degree of personal distress and impairment.

Collecting as a hobby and hoarding as a psychiatric disorder share certain similarities, but there is a significant difference between these two activities. A hobbyist collector usually takes pleasure in acquiring specific items that hold personal interest or value, such as stamps, coins, or antique cars and furniture. They typically display their collection in an organized manner, maintain it properly, and are often eager to share their collection with others, showcasing a sense of pride and accomplishment. Their collecting habits do not interfere with their daily lives, relationships, or living spaces.

Hoarding, on the other hand, is a recognized psychiatric disorder characterized by an excessive accumulation of items, regardless of their actual value or usefulness. Their belongings typically clutter their living spaces, making it difficult to use rooms for their intended purposes. This behavior often leads to significant distress, impairment in functioning, and can even pose risks to health or safety. For instance, a person hoarding newspapers might fill their entire house with stacks of old papers, to the point where navigating through the house becomes challenging.

One of my earliest patients was a hoarder of newspapers. I asked him why he did it. He replied that he might miss some important news if he threw away the newspapers. I tired persuasion, arguing that once he finished reading the newspaper, he would have digested all the news, so there would be nothing to "miss." My argument held no sway. Similar to a person with obsessive-compulsive disorder (OCD), he recognized his behavior was irrational, but he was helpless in overcoming it. I had to refer him to a psychologist who specialized in treating patients with OCD.

While it might seem like a fine line between collecting and hoarding, the two are distinguishable by the purpose, organization, and impact of the behavior. Collecting brings joy and satisfaction, whereas hoarding often results in distress and functional impairment. Unlike hoarders, collectors typically do not struggle to part with any of their possessions, especially if paid for their collection. Collectors usually do not perceive an intense need to save their items. There are exceptions, of course, and I am one of them.

I have been collecting compact discs (CDs) since they were commercially released in the mid-1980s. Much of my collection, however, consists of live concerts that were never commercially released—they were aired live (e.g., on the radio), tape-recorded, and then digitized by music lovers all over the world. The concerts were made available for downloading on certain websites that usually only music lovers knew about. These concerts were known as recordings of independent origin (ROIO); they were never copyrighted, so people like me felt free to download them for their own enjoyment and burn them on blank discs, unless of course the artists explicitly prohibited it and invoked the Digital Millennium Copyright Act. However, many musicians encouraged free downloading of their music, most notably, the Grateful Dead.

Recently, I was forced to abandon thousands of CDs because I moved and downsized my primary residence. My dilemma was how to decide which CDs to save (I could only bring a few hundred to the new home). What would be my internal algorithm for saving CDs versus discarding them? It was a very difficult and painful process, yet not entirely alien to me. Soon after I began collecting CDs I could tell it was becoming a borderline obsession. I discussed it with my analyst, but he confessed he was suffering a similar problem—collecting books!

Apparently, neither of us was alone in our struggle to limit our collection. My narrative medicine instructor informed me about an Irish historian who hosted peace and reconciliation workshops following the "Troubles." This individual had one of the largest collections of Irish books. He sold his pub on the sole condition that after his death his ashes remain in perpetuity by the doorway of the pub that housed his books. What an extreme example of how people who are genuinely into collecting—not hoarding—find it difficult to part with their possessions.

My instructor further commented, "I have observed how my little collections comfort me until I'm ready to let them go. My car is never tidy, but whenever my daughter needed a sweater, other shoes, water, snacks, and often more off-the-wall items, I could say, 'I think there's one in the back.' And there was. I think [collecting] is a leftover practice from our roaming hominid days. Sometimes maladaptive and often delightful."

Indeed, the act of collecting can be viewed as an evolutionary behavior that dates back to our early ancestors. It may have originally served a survival function, as early hominids gathered resources such as food, tools, and materials for shelter. This instinct to gather and store has persisted into the modern era, manifesting in the form of collecting behaviors.

Collecting, in its healthy form, can certainly be a delightful practice. It can provide a sense of accomplishment and satisfaction, offer an avenue for relaxation and enjoyment, and even foster social connections through shared interests. Collectors relish in their collections, which may reflect their personal interests, experiences, or values. I have come across doctors whose collections have varied from renown racing cars to prestigious bottles of wine.

However, like any behavior, collecting can become maladaptive when it becomes excessive or obsessive, interfering with a person's daily life and well-being. This is where the line between collecting and hoarding is drawn. While collecting may indeed be a "leftover practice from our roaming hominid days," it is crucial to recognize when this behavior crosses the line from a delightful hobby to a psychiatric hoarding disorder. It is important to make this distinction to ensure those who are hoarding receive the necessary mental health help and support.

38

Further Musings on Collecting and Hoarding

Online exchanges while pruning my CDs.

Surgeon: Art, I've given some thought to your remarks about collecting versus hoarding. When I retired, nine years ago, I methodically went through a stash of boxes from our last move (never unpacked—that tells you something about their contents) and got rid of a lot of stuff. I also thought seriously about downsizing—what would I take with me, what would I leave? By the end of a year or so, all the boxes were gone and most everything in our house had a mental tag on it.

But then we decided that we were going to stay in our house, which is a large house (not a McMansion, but a good size) and that removed the necessity to discard stuff. I seem to have heard somewhere that all those old English country houses are full of stuff that nobody bothered to discard. Accumulated because there was space.

Many years ago, I hosted a visiting professor from the surgery dept. at [a well-known medical school]. He lived in a tiny apartment. He wanted me to show him the flea markets. What could he possibly collect in such a small space? He told me he collected "paper"— old deeds, and so on—things of little intrinsic value that were meaningful to him. We went to four or five flea markets and I don't think he bought anything. How does the shape of the space we inhabit influence our habits?

[My husband] and I both grew up hearing tales of the Great Depression at the dinner table. It shaped the arc of our parents' lives. We were taught not to waste anything. I still mend clothes, rather than discarding them. Partly it is because old clothes are more comfortable than new. Still, I wonder if this is a generational thing? 'Generational trauma?' I hesitate to use the term because even at the height of the Great Depression, our families were never in danger of starving.

Me: My dad grew up during the Great Depression. He attributed his morbid obesity to the fact that he always ate everything on his plate—whether he was hungry or not—because he never knew where his next meal would come from. He rationalized his behavior, but there was some truth to what he said. Notably, he was not a collector of anything.

Surgeon: When I throw things out, not even Goodwill wants them... Slight exaggeration.

Me: I am on the "S" section of my CDs. My formula has been to discard commercially released material—I have most of that stored digitally—and keep the best of the live concerts broadcast on-air but never officially released on CD. If there are too many from one artist, my next "cutoff" is to keep only CDs recorded at venues in cities that were special to my travels, mainly Boston and Philly (college and med school/hometown). I should have mentioned that I also have several hundred DVD concerts, commercial and 'bootleg.' I'm keeping those! Not to mention that there is so much music on YouTube for the taking (with proper software). In a few months, I'll have forgotten what I threw out, which is ultimate proof of its lack of utility. The main difference between hoarding and collecting lies in the degree of impairment and personal distress caused by the former. Dr. Robert Spitzer, the 'father' of psychiatric nosology and main architect of the groundbreaking DSM-III, put forth the idea that ultimately what defines a mental disorder is functional impairment and distress. I think most of us 'collectors' are on safe ground!

My narrative medicine instructor chimed in to our online conversation.

Instructor: Art. I deeply appreciate your sensitivity to a hoarder's process. The phrase 'letting go' gets tossed about without respect to ways we each cope with the material world. Every object has a story, some kind of marker for possible meaning. We all know we are missing half (at least) of the whole picture. If we don't know what we are seeking how do we know where to look until the giant cosmic flashlight illuminates?

This is a beautiful quote I read (about hoarding):

'If a family member just went in and removed the clutter it would most likely result in disastrous consequences, including: rupture of trust, alienating the family member, increasing the family member's anxiety, depression/suicidality, thus potentially delaying their time to receiving care and treatment.'

Of course, this is coming from a kid whose bedroom got so full and messy, I moved into a tent by the sea wall. I didn't face my room until a severe tropical storm lifted my tent with me in it. For some it takes an act of God.

Me: Perhaps a higher power is involved in some way, if not in giving up items, at least in collecting them. Some individuals may hoard items due to beliefs related to material wealth, preservation of resources, or the sacredness of certain objects. For others, hoarding may be linked to fears of death or loss. The act of accumulating items can create a sense of control and security, which may help to alleviate underlying fears or insecurities related to morbidity and mortality.

Over time, I framed my diplomas, educational certificates, and professional awards. Within a few decades, the number had grown to nearly two-dozen. What to do with them? I couldn't hang all of them on my office wall—there wasn't enough space, and it would appear too gaudy. Yet, I didn't want to part with them. I asked my analyst for suggestions.

"Art," he said, "you'll know which ones to keep."

Now, in my 70s, I do indeed know which ones to keep—only a fraction—and I removed them from their frames. The parchments are safely stored with a few of my other precious belongings. I would like some tangible evidence of my accomplishments for my children and especially my grandchildren to remember me by.

39

Why do Physicians—and Psychiatrists in Particular—Write?

Hint: It's not for the money!

All writers want recognition of some sort. No?

Recognition can take many forms, such as positive feedback, awards, or simply the knowledge that their work is being read and appreciated. However, it is important to note that motivation can vary among writers. Some may write primarily for personal satisfaction, to express themselves, or to contribute to a specific field or cause.

Some writers write to make a living. In fact, professional writing can be a lucrative career. This includes a broad range of fields, such as journalism, content creation, technical writing, and editing, among others. But as a friend reminded me, "Not even the greats like Eliot, Hardy, Pound, and Yeats ever got rich writing. Whatever they made, they blew on whiskey, women, and snuff"—and they were not alone.

In the context of health care, medical writers often work for pharmaceutical companies, research institutions, or medical publications. Their work can involve creating content for educational materials, research papers, regulatory documents, and promotional literature. The compensation they receive can vary greatly depending on their level of expertise, the complexity of the task, and the organization they work for.

Why do Physicians Write?

In my experience, the primary drive for most physician writers is to make a positive impact in their profession and for their patients—not necessarily for recognition, income, or to pen a bestseller. Writing allows physicians to reach a larger audience beyond their own practice and influence health care on a broader scale. Their primary motivation often lies in the advancement of health care and the betterment of patient outcomes.

Physicians possess vast amounts of knowledge and experience in their respective fields, and writing provides an avenue to share this information on a larger scale. For example, a doctor specializing in cardiovascular health might choose to write articles or books about preventing heart disease, or a business-minded physician might write to give advice on personal finance.

Additionally, writing serves as a tool for education. Physicians can use their writings to educate other health care professionals, students, and even the general public on a variety of health-related topics. For instance, a pediatrician might write a comprehensive guide on the importance of childhood vaccinations to help parents understand their significance.

Writing also contributes to the advancement of medicine. Physicians can write about their research findings or clinical experiences to help push the field forward. An oncologist, for example, might publish a paper about new treatment approaches for a specific type of cancer.

Advocacy is another motivation for physicians to write. They can use their writings to advocate for changes in health policy or to raise awareness about specific health issues. A physician working in a low-resource setting might write articles or op-eds to highlight the need for better health care infrastructure.

Many physicians (like me) also write as a form of reflective practice. They might write personal essays or narratives about their interactions with patients, bringing a more humanistic perspective to the medical profession. Their writing contributes to the broader field of narrative medicine and often reflects the emotional and physical health benefits of expressive writing.

Writing also serves as a means of patient education. Physicians can write blog posts on common health questions, create patient information leaflets, or even write books about managing specific health conditions.

Lastly, writing can contribute to a physician's professional development. By publishing in peer-reviewed journals or reputable health websites, they can demonstrate their expertise and knowledge in their field.

Who do Psychiatrists Write?

Psychiatrists, like other physicians, are often motivated to write to share their knowledge, educate others, contribute to the progression of their field, and advocate for their patients. However, psychiatry's unique focus on the complex world of mental health introduces certain specific influences on their motivations and the style of their narratives.

Psychiatry fundamentally revolves around understanding the human mind. Psychiatrists' writings are likely to delve deeper into the exploration of emotions, thoughts, and behaviors. The act of writing, especially in a reflective or narrative style, allows psychiatrists to articulate their insights about human behavior, feelings, and relationships.

Their narratives might also contain more discussions of societal and cultural factors, as these aspects significantly influence mental health. Furthermore, the therapeutic relationship between the doctor and patient, a central component of psychiatric treatment, is often a prominent theme in psychiatrists' narratives.

Because psychiatry often deals with intricate and deeply personal patient stories, writing provides psychiatrists with a platform to share these compelling narratives while preserving patient confidentiality. This not only helps educate others about mental health but also works towards reducing associated stigmas.

The emotionally intense nature of their work also makes writing a valuable tool for psychiatrists for reflection and self-care. It offers a therapeutic outlet and a means to process the emotional aspects of their profession.

Another significant motivator for psychiatrists to write is advocacy, as mentioned above. The field of mental health has historically faced issues of underfunding and stigmatization. Writing becomes a powerful means for psychiatrists to raise awareness about mental health issues and advocate for policy changes.

Writing also serves as an effective way for psychiatrists to educate patients and their families. They can write about different mental health conditions, treatment options, and strategies for managing mental health. The demand for self-help and self-improvement books and articles is quite high. One study estimates the worth of the global self-improvement market size and share at $81.6 billion by 2032.

Regardless, the act of writing allows all physicians to educate, advocate, reflect, and contribute to the field of medicine with the ultimate aim of improving patient care and health outcomes and contributing to a better understanding of the human condition.

40

Scams Perpetrated on Physician Authors by Impersonators and Bad Actors

There is a high prevalence of fraud and other bad practices in and around the publishing industry.

There are millions of scams every year impacting individuals of all backgrounds, in every corner of the world, and with novel and changing techniques and lures. Categories include: products and services, charity, phantom debt, prize and grant, relationship and trust, employment, and investment. Criminals target different populations for each type of fraud, with physicians most often falling victim to investment fraud.

Increasingly, however, doctors and other type of healthcare providers are becoming victims of publishing scams, a subtype of "products and services" scams. Because so many doctors are writing and publishing these days, they should be alert for it.

As a matter of fact, shortly after publishing a book, I received what seemed like a promising film adaptation offer from a reputable-sounding company. Despite initial excitement, I discovered it was a sophisticated scam. This experience taught me to stay vigilant and verify unsolicited offers—not only book and movie deals, but any business promise that appeals to your ego and seems like a get-rich-quick scheme.

Many accounts similar to mine have been reported on the internet. One of the best articles I found was published in *Medical Economics* in 2016, titled 6 Reasons Doctors Get Scammed. The article was written by James M. Dahle, MD, founder of the "White Coat Investor." Dr Dahle hosts the most widely-read, physician-specific personal finance and investing website in the world. You would be grossly mistaken to think that smart doctors and other medical professionals are not susceptible to fraud.

According to Dr. Dahle, doctors get scammed frequently. They are targeted due to their naivety, trust in professionals, lack of sophistication, and especially high incomes. In addition, they are poorly trained in business, too busy to do proper due diligence, and overconfident, often failing to heed even the basic principles of investing. Some physicians misplace their trust in "friends of friends," and others simply harbor a "fear of missing out" (FOMO).

To avoid being conned, Dr. Dahle recommends that physicians learn about finance, obtain second opinions from independent advisors, and pass on "fishy" investment opportunities. I have additional recommendations for physician writers—indeed, creatives in general—that might help them avoid publishing scams. My recommendations have been adapted from the official blog of Writer Beware® by Victoria Strauss, an author on a mission "[to] shine a bright light into the dark corners of the shadow-world of literary scams, schemes, and pitfalls."

Here are some of her tips and mine:

1. **Verify Identities:** Always verify the identities of individuals and companies making unsolicited offers. Cross-check their contact details and credentials through official channels. Hundreds of bona fide entities have been skillfully impersonated by bad actors representing movie companies, producers, agents, publishers, bookstores, and media companies.

2. **Consult Professionals:** If approached with offers involving significant rights or financial transactions, consult with a literary agent or legal professional before proceeding.

3. **Ask for a Reality Check:** Don't forget the adage that if something is too good to be true it probably is. It's difficult to be objective about your own work, so seek the opinions of family members and trusted colleagues who don't have skin in the game. Ask them for an honest opinion whether the offer seems real or fake and what makes your work so special that it would be singled out among a thousand others also deserving recognition.

4. **Check Your Ego:** While it's natural to feel flattered by interest in your work, it's essential to stay grounded. Scammers often exploit pride and excitement, so approach such offers with a healthy dose of skepticism. Remember that legitimate opportunities usually come through established channels and often involve due diligence and formal processes.

5. **Beware Foreign Actors:** At present, most scams impacting U.S.-based writers come from overseas—the Philippines, Pakistan and India. They are highly predatory and may be linked to so-called "vanity publishers" using overseas employees to produce your work. It's a risk that authors take when they self-publish their writing.

6. **Keep an Eye on Your Finances:** Scammers will try to hook you and pressure you to spend money on goods and services that may be highly overpriced, non-existent, never actually delivered, or all three. Some have the means (through leaked information) to access your online banking information and hack your account. Never provide your bank account and routing numbers to anyone other than the most trusted authorities. Do *not* share your bank information with

your publisher unless proper fraud precautions have been established—such as in a real estate wiring transaction.

7. **Remain Skeptical of Unsolicited Offers:** Scammers primarily acquire sensitive information by phishing through solicitation, and they are persistent. It is extremely rare for reputable business people to contact authors out of the blue, although it sometimes happens. Rule number one to protect yourself from a scam is never give your personal information over the phone.

8. **Reject Purchase Fees and Requirements:** Reputable agents, publishers, and production companies should not charge you for their representation or rights to acquire your work. Do not let them sell you any type of service, or refer you to any third-party company or provider you have to pay.

9. **Report Suspicious Activity:** Report any suspicious offers or communications to relevant authorities or industry bodies to help protect others from similar scams. Write or talk about your experience and warn your writing group or close associates to be careful and avoid these scams. Speak up against those who have committed financial crimes (only 14% are reported to the police). You may not recover your money if you have been scammed, but you can protect others from becoming victims.

10. **Expect Professionalism at All Times:** Whether you are approached in writing or through a telephone call, watch out for these additional tell-tale signs. They are highly correlated with author scams:

    o   Form letters, mismatched fonts, pasted material, and other examples that lack personalized communication

- o Spoofed phone numbers and addresses that do not match the location of the company that the individual claims to represent
- o Suspicious emails: misspellings; grammatical errors; threatening with consequences; requesting personal information and/or user IDs; dubious links; offering fantastic prizes; creating a sense of urgency
- o Over-the-top compliments and flattering and flowery praise of your work
- o Overly-friendly first lines or presumptive acquaintances ("I hope this email finds you in good health and high spirits and that you are still thriving in your personal journey.")
- o A guarantee that your work has been thoroughly read and vetted by—or recommended to—company executives
- o Evidence of English as a second language, or use of pronunciation applications for non-native English speakers, e.g., BoldVoice

My fifth-grade teacher often said, "A word to the wise is sufficient," as she would admonish a student and set them straight. She believed that once warned, the student's wayward behavior would not recur. By sharing my experience, I aim to raise awareness among fellow authors and creatives, helping them avoid the scams that I have encountered.

Authors, let this be your "word."

The Power of "Enough-ness" in Medicine

How the principles of "Dayenu" apply in everyday practice

My son, his wife, and their 3-year-old son made the long flight from their home in Honolulu to our "summer" home in Asheville, North Carolina, a charming town situated in the foothills of the Blue Ridge Mountains. Normally, my wife and I make the trek to Honolulu twice a year to visit them. However, this time, we were spared a visit (expense), and in doing so, we were able to have a large family and friends gathering.

After their visit, and as I dropped off my son at the airport, I looked at him intently and said, "You know, your mother and I would have met you half-way. It would have been enough for you to fly to the west coast and meet us there rather than schlep to Asheville."

My son immediately invoked the Hebrew term "Dayenu" (pronounced "die-yay-new"). "Dayenu" translates to "it would have been enough" in English. "Dayenu" is both an expression and a song. The latter consists of 15 stanzas referencing different historical contexts the Israelites experienced during slavery in Egypt. It is traditionally sung on Passover to express gratitude for each of the many gifts that God bestowed to the Jewish people during their exodus from Egypt, stating that each act in itself would have been enough.

While "Dayenu" originates from a religious context, its underlying principles can offer valuable secular lessons, even in health care.

Applying the concept of "Dayenu" to the practice of medicine may seem "unorthodox," but it can manifest in various ways. One instance is in patient care, where physicians can encourage patients to adopt an attitude of gratitude for any progress they make in their health journey, regardless of the size. This can contribute to patient satisfaction and overall mental well-being, which can also positively affect their physical health.

The concept of "Dayenu" can help physicians appreciate their achievements and the progress they've made in their career or in treating a patient, even if they haven't reached the end goal. Healthcare providers can find solace in each small improvement in a patient's condition. Celebrating small victories can boost the morale of physicians, helping to mitigate burnout, which is arguably the most plaguing issue in the medical profession today.

As "Dayenu" (the song) builds, it calls out miracles, punctuating each one with *Dayenu!* The song's structure, which highlights a series of incremental steps, parallels the step-by-step approach often needed in medical treatment and recovery. Understanding that each small improvement is significant can help manage expectations and maintain motivation in long-term care or complex medical situations.

"Dayenu" teaches the importance of seeing the broader picture while recognizing the value of individual components. In medicine, this can translate to a holistic approach to patient care, where addressing physical, emotional, and psychological aspects of health are all deemed important.

The principles of sufficiency and contentment inherent in "Dayenu" can prompt healthcare providers to reflect on ethical issues such as the limits of intervention, resource allocation, and the balance between aggressive treatment and quality of life. Specifically, the principle of "Dayenu" aligns with the idea of avoiding overtreatment in medical interventions. This approach recognizes when enough has been done for a patient's health, understanding that further intervention may not improve, and could potentially harm, the patient's quality of life.

The historical context of "Dayenu" is one of overcoming adversity and oppression. In medicine, maintaining resilience and hope is crucial for both patients facing difficult diagnoses and for healthcare workers managing the demands of their profession. The song's message can be a source of inspiration and strength for everyone.

Indeed, "Dayenu" was used to explain the final game of the 2016 World Series that gave the Chicago Cubs a win after 108 years of drought. Just as "Dayenu" teaches the importance of recognizing and appreciating each blessing, the Cubs' historic journey to their World Series win encourages fans to appreciate each moment and milestone that contributed to their ultimate triumph.

In essence, the values represented by "Dayenu"—gratitude, contentment, and moderation—originating from a specific religious tradition can be universally applied, including within the field of medicine. By drawing lessons from this ancient song, healthcare professionals can enhance their practice, ensuring they not only treat illnesses but also nurture the overall well-being of their patients.

42

Issues Involved in Making Informed Medical Decisions

Always consider the "X factor" and never take your health for granted.

During a routine visit with my primary care physician (PCP) I complained about feeling fatigued. My general health is good, but my PCP suggested checking my thyroid levels as well as B12 and testosterone. The results came back normal except for testosterone. My overall testosterone level was normal, but my free testosterone was mildly low at 6.2 (normal is between 6.6 - 18.1 pg/mL). My PCP messaged me that if I have any interest in replacement therapy to just let him know.

I should let him know? Isn't it his job to determine whether therapy is necessary? Is this what we mean by patient-centered care—let the decisions fall to the patient? Or maybe because I *am* a physician my PCP assumed I knew as much (or more) about testosterone replacement therapy than he did.

The response from my PCP was perplexing. It highlights several crucial aspects about patient independence, mutual decision-making, the interaction between healthcare professionals, and knowledge of evidence-based treatment. Let's parse out some of these issues in order to examine some of the components of *informed* decision-making.

Patient Autonomy and Shared Decision-Making. The concept of patient autonomy and shared decision-making comes into play with my PCP's suggestion about replacement therapy and leaving the decision to me. This is a fundamental part of patient-centric care, where patients are actively involved in their care decisions. It's not about passing all decisions to the patient, but rather engaging them in the decision-making process, considering their values, preferences, and needs.

Communication Through Health Portals. My doctor may have suggested replacement therapy as an option because my free testosterone was only mildly low and perhaps he didn't see it as immediately necessary, but was open to considering it if I felt strongly about it. I don't know if this was the case because communication through health portals can sometimes be limiting and may contribute to misunderstandings or assumptions. In face-to-face consultations, physicians can use visual cues, tone of voice, and body language to better gauge a patient's understanding or concerns, and patients can immediately ask questions. This dynamic is altered in written communication via health portals.

Role of the Physician. While it is ostensibly the duty of my PCP to determine if therapy is necessary, it doesn't mean he should make all the decisions independently. The role of a doctor is to offer the best possible advice based on medical knowledge and experience. However, the ultimate decision often rests with the patient, after they've been thoroughly informed about the benefits, risks, and alternatives. Again, this represents another shortcoming of messaging through internet channels: messages must be brief due to the nature of the communication medium and time limitations imposed upon healthcare professionals to fully explain the pros and cons of a potential treatment.

Relationship Between Healthcare Professionals: Being a physician myself might have influenced the way my PCP communicated with me. He might have assumed that I have a deeper understanding of my health and the implications of different treatment paths. However, this assumption may not always be accurate or fair, as physicians also need straightforward guidance when they are the patients.

Practice Guidelines and Evidence-Based Treatment. It is possible that my PCP might have left the choice to me, assuming I would do my own research or already have the knowledge to make an informed decision. Given the borderline nature of my results and the potential risks and benefits of testosterone therapy, my personal input as a knowledgeable patient would be valuable. While practice guidelines and evidence-based treatment provide a foundation for care, they do not eliminate the need for individual clinical judgment, patient preferences, and shared decision-making. This is particularly relevant in scenarios like mine, where the best course of action may not be clearly defined by the guidelines.

Self-Treatment. The adage "A doctor who treats himself has a fool for a patient" emphasizes the potential pitfalls of self-diagnosis and treatment. It suggests that even physicians can have blind spots when it comes to their own health, and that it is important to seek an objective, outside perspective. This is vital because personal bias or emotional involvement can cloud judgment, potentially leading to misdiagnosis or inappropriate treatment. This includes advice from family members who are medical professionals.

Repeat Testing. Lab tests are not always 100% accurate. There can be errors, contamination, or even a simple mix-up. Repeat testing helps to confirm that the initial results were correct. Hormone levels, like testosterone, can fluctuate throughout the day and can be influenced by various factors such as diet, stress, sleep, and physical activity. Especially in cases where treatment might have significant side effects, it's crucial to be certain that treatment is necessary. Repeat testing can provide this certainty.

The "X Factor." The term "X factor" generally refers to an unknown, variable, or unpredictable element or factor that could have a significant impact on the outcome of a situation. In the context of a medical case, the "X factor" could refer to an unknown aspect of a patient's condition, an underlying disease, a genetic factor, an environmental factor, or even a patient's personal habits or lifestyle that might be influencing their health. As it might apply to a case with equivocal lab results, the "X factor" could be a potential reason why the results are borderline. Identifying and understanding this "X factor" could be key to determining the best course of treatment.

Ultimately, I decided to forgo therapy. There were several reasons for my decision. First, the American Urological Association guidelines recommend treatment only when the total testosterone level is below 300 ng/dL (mine was 378 ng/dL). Second, it is quite possible that my fatigue is related to obstructive sleep apnea, a confirmed diagnosis yet one whose primary treatment—continuous positive airway pressure—is difficult for me to tolerate. Third, I was not keen on receiving hormone therapy in light of my history of depression. Lastly, there are lingering concerns about the side effects of testosterone therapy, mainly surrounding prostate cancer development and cardiovascular events.

I've only attempted to outline the very basic issues surrounding informed medical decision-making. Although it is vital to maintain open communication with your PCP, if you feel puzzled or unsure about any aspect of your care, it's important to express that and seek further information. If you're uncertain about the need for any type of therapy, you should discuss the potential benefits and risks with your PCP *in person* to make an informed decision. Always seek clarification when in doubt and never take your health for granted.

43

Doctors, Heed Your Parents' Advice

*Famous sayings of fictional moms and dads
and their relevance to medical practice.*

Forrest Gump's and Bobby Boucher's mothers gained fame through the movies *Forrest Gump* and *The Waterboy*, with Tom Hanks and Adam Sandler playing the lead roles and Sally Field and Kathy Bates portraying their mothers. These characters offered a wealth of practical advice that, while not originally intended for medical professionals, holds special significance for doctors.

Here are a few examples of the practical advice given by Forrest Gump's and Bobby Boucher's mothers, along with their potential significance for doctors:

1. **Forrest Gump's Mama: "Life is like a box of chocolates. You never know what you're gonna get."**
   o *Significance for Doctors:* This saying can remind doctors that each patient is unique and that they should be prepared for a variety of outcomes and challenges in their practice. It emphasizes the importance of being adaptable and open-minded.

2. **Forrest Gump's Mama: "Stupid is as stupid does."**
   o *Significance for Doctors:* This underscores the importance of actions and decisions in defining a physician's competence and character. It serves as a reminder that what truly matters is how physicians

apply their knowledge, interact with patients and colleagues, and uphold professional standards in their daily practice.

3. **Forrest Gump's Mama: "You have to do the best with what God gave you."**
   - *Significance for Doctors:* This encourages acceptance and making the most out of any situation. It can remind doctors to provide the best possible care with the resources available and to encourage patients to focus on their strengths and capabilities.

4. **Bobby Boucher's Mama: "Foosball is the devil!"**
   - *Significance for Doctors:* While humorous and exaggerated, this line can serve as a reminder that misinformation and personal biases can affect decision-making. Doctors need to rely on scientific evidence and critical thinking rather than myths, misconceptions, or disinformation.

5. **Bobby Boucher's Mama: "You can do it!"**
   - *Significance for Doctors:* This encouragement can be seen as a reminder of the importance of support and motivation in patient care. Physicians should strive to empower their patients, providing encouragement and reassurance, especially during challenging treatments or recovery periods. "You can do it!" can also be a powerful motivator for doctors and encourage them to strive for the highest levels of leadership in their career.

These examples illustrate how the practical advice given by the characters' mothers, though not originally intended for the medical field, can hold valuable lessons for doctors in their everyday practice.

Here are a few other famous "mamas" from movies and literature, their notable sayings, and the implications for doctors or medical practice:

6. **Molly Weasley (*Harry Potter and the Deathly Hallows* by J.K Rowling): "Not my daughter, you bitch!"**
   - *Significance for Doctors:* This powerful statement of protection and advocacy can remind doctors of the importance of fiercely advocating for their patients, especially in situations where their well-being might be threatened.

7. **Leigh Anne Tuohy (Sandra Bullock) (*The Blind Side*): "You threaten my son, you threaten me."**
   - *Significance for Doctors:* This shows the importance of a strong support system for patients. Doctors should recognize the role of family and caregivers in the healing process and work collaboratively with them. It can also serve as a call to doctors and families to vehemently fight adverse decisions made by insurance companies that deny patients necessary medical care.

8. **Amy March (*Little Women* by Louisa May Alcott): "I am not afraid of storms, for I am learning how to sail my ship."**
   - **Significance for Doctors:** This can be a metaphor for resilience and continuous learning. Physicians should embrace challenges and view them as opportunities for growth and learning, both personally and professionally.

9. **Aurora Greenway (Shirley MacLaine) (*Terms of Endearment*): "I just want you to know, I'm a very stubborn woman."**
   - *Significance for Doctors:* This highlights the importance of perseverance and determination. For doctors, it suggests the need to be persistent in seeking the

best outcomes for their patients, even in the face of adversity.

10. **Sarah Connor (Linda Hamilton) (*Terminator 2: Judgment Day*): "There is no fate but what we make for ourselves."**
    - ○ *Significance for Doctors*: This can be interpreted as a call to proactive and preventative care. Doctors can use this to underscore the importance of patient empowerment and preventive health measures, emphasizing that patients have a significant role in shaping their health outcomes.

These examples illustrate how the wisdom of fictional mothers can impart valuable lessons for medical professionals, encouraging qualities such as advocacy, resilience, support, perseverance, and proactive care.

But what about dads? Are there any famous dads from movies and novels whose notable sayings may have relevance to doctors or medical practice? Here are a few that come to mind:

11. **Atticus Finch (Gregory Peck) (*To Kill a Mockingbird*): "You never really understand a person until you consider things from his point of view...Until you climb inside of his skin and walk around in it."**
    - ○ Significance for Doctors: This emphasizes the importance of empathy in medical practice. Doctors should strive to understand their patients' perspectives and experiences to provide compassionate and effective care.

12. **Mufasa (James Earl Jones) (*The Lion King*): "Remember who you are."**
    - ○ *Significance for Doctors:* This can be a reminder for doctors to stay true to their values, ethics, and the principles of medical practice. It underscores the

importance of integrity and self-awareness in the profession.

13. **Vito Corleone (Marlon Brando) (*The Godfather*): "A man who doesn't spend time with his family can never be a real man."**
    o *Significance for Doctors:* This can serve as a reminder of the importance of work-life balance. Doctors should ensure they make time for their families and personal lives to maintain their own well-being and prevent burnout.

14. **Daniel Hillard (Robin Williams) (*Mrs. Doubtfire*): "If there's love, dear... those are the ties that bind, and you'll have a family in your heart, forever."**
    o *Significance for Doctors:* This emphasizes the importance of love and compassion. In medical practice, maintaining a compassionate approach to patient care can strengthen the doctor-patient relationship and improve patient outcomes.

15. **Chris Gardner (Will Smith) (*The Pursuit of Happyness*): "You got a dream... You gotta protect it. People can't do something themselves, they wanna tell you you can't do it. If you want something, go get it. Period."**
    o *Significance for Doctors:* This is a powerful message about determination and pursuing one's goals. For doctors, it underscores the importance of dedication to their profession and their continuous pursuit of excellence in patient care and personal development.

16. **Arthur Weasley (*Harry Potter and the Chamber of Secrets* by J.K. Rowling): "Never trust anything that can think for itself if you can't see where it keeps its brain."**
    o *Significance for Doctors:* This can be a cautionary reminder about the reliance on technology, automated

systems, and artificial intelligence in medicine. Doctors should always apply critical thinking and not blindly trust technology without understanding its limitations and implications.

These examples illustrate how the wisdom of fictional fathers can impart valuable lessons for medical professionals, encouraging qualities such as empathy, perseverance, integrity, work-life balance, compassion, determination, and critical thinking.

Lastly, let's not forget:

17. **Arnold Schwarzenegger (*The Terminator*): "I'll be back."**
    o *Significance for Doctors:* This phrase can symbolize reliability and follow-through. For doctors, it emphasizes the importance of continuity of care and the commitment to their patients. It is a reminder that doctors should always make an effort to check on their patients, follow up on treatments, and ensure ongoing support and care. It builds trust and reassures patients that their doctor is dedicated to their long-term health.

By drawing inspiration from this and other memorable lines, physicians can reinforce their dedication to patient care and the importance of being consistently present and available for their patients.

44

Observations on Healthcare Leadership

Despite the clear differences between physicians and business executives, both must possess qualities that can drive change—and lead to its acceptance.

Although my journey has included practicing medicine, leading teams, attending business school, working in health insurance and pharma, and consulting, the core focus of my work has always remained the same: improving the health of individuals served by the companies I worked and consulted for. At heart, I am still a clinician.

I currently consult for several healthcare organizations. People frequently ask how I transitioned from a full-time psychiatry practice to assisting healthcare companies and their leaders in managing their clinical operations.

Whereas I once focused directly on patients and their families, I now support them indirectly by collaborating with leaders and their organizations. You might say that my "H&P" (history and physical) now includes not only patients but also organizational structures, habits, beliefs, and relationships. These insights help my clients gain a comprehensive understanding of the current state of population health and refine their patient improvement initiatives.

Effective organizational change requires time and deliberate effort, but through this process, clients develop organizational trust, competency, and leadership capacity. Transitioning from caring for patients and their families to aiding healthcare organizations in their success, I continue to love what I do. The continuous theme of helping people and the systems they belong to seamlessly ties together this unique career path.

However, working with organizational leaders who are not medically trained is not easy. It requires patience and an understanding of their psychological makeup. The Myers-Briggs Type Inventory (MBTI) has shown that physicians and non-physician CEOs have virtually polar opposite personalities, yet there are remarkable similarities in the personality traits of non-physician healthcare executives and general business CEOs.

Psychological processes likely play a significant role in shaping the communication patterns and relationships within healthcare organizations. Understanding the essential psychological differences among individuals can provide physicians with valuable insights into the thoughts and behaviors of their nonmedical colleagues. This understanding, combined with the motivation to act on it, can significantly enhance relationships, particularly through improved communication.

Given that individual psychological preferences are crucial to the communication process and often differ greatly between physicians and non-physician executives, there is an opportunity to enhance communication by tailoring it to these preferences. Developing a "common language" can help foster better relationships between physicians and business leaders.

In addition to personality and communication differences, physicians and non-physician executives frequently exhibit distinct interaction and leadership styles. These variations stem from their specialized training, professional experiences, and differing organizational roles and responsibilities.

Physicians typically have extensive clinical training, focusing on patient care, diagnosis, and treatment. Their decision-making is usually grounded in clinical evidence, patient outcomes, and medical ethics. They often work in hierarchical healthcare teams, leading clinical decisions while collaborating closely with other healthcare professionals like nurses and technicians.

In contrast, non-physician executives usually come from backgrounds in business, management, finance, or administration. Their decisions tend to be driven by organizational strategy, financial performance, and operational efficiency. They lead through management structures, emphasizing broader organizational goals, resource allocation, and strategic planning.

When it comes to leadership styles, physicians often have a high degree of autonomy in clinical settings and may be used to making decisions independently or with minimal input from others. Their leadership style is typically rooted in evidence-based practices and a deep understanding of medical science, with a strong focus on patient care and outcomes.

Non-physician executives, on the other hand, may employ more collaborative and inclusive leadership styles, engaging various stakeholders in decision-making processes. They focus on long-term strategic goals, organizational growth, and sustainability, with a strong emphasis on efficiency, cost-effectiveness, and resource management.

In terms of interaction styles, physicians often center their interactions around clinical issues, patient care discussions, and medical problem-solving. They might be more accustomed to interacting within a hierarchical framework, especially in clinical settings.

Non-physician executives, however, center their interactions around organizational performance, strategic initiatives, and business operations. They tend to engage with a wide range of departments and functions, fostering cross-functional collaboration and communication.

Physicians may face challenges when transitioning to broader organizational leadership roles that require business acumen and strategic thinking. Many, like myself, have sought an MBA degree to fill the void. Business training, coupled with physicians' deep understanding of clinical operations and patient care, can provide valuable insights for improving healthcare delivery and patient outcomes.

Non-physician executives might encounter difficulties in understanding the complexities of clinical decision-making and patient care dynamics. It is extremely rare for them to go—or want to go—to medical school after completing business school. Nevertheless, the expertise of non-physician executives in management and strategy can drive organizational efficiency, financial stability, and innovation in healthcare delivery.

One of the most frequent errors made by both physician and non-physician leaders is underestimating the effort required to implement clinical changes. Prioritizing speed over thoroughness often leads to subpar outcomes, and organizations generally underperform when they compromise quality for rapid execution. Adopting a Wall Street-driven approach is even more detrimental and can lead to complete business failure.

Additionally, what might appear to be a minor adjustment to current practices often triggers anger, resentment, backlash, and resistance to change. Leaders can be caught off guard by such reactions, unaware that a deep-rooted system maintains the status quo and resists change. These roots are substantial. Even if dysfunctional, the existing systems, processes, and norms have developed for specific reasons; they are not random but rather a reflection of the people who work there.

Taking the time to understand the culture that established the status quo, considering what change might signify for individuals, and helping them recognize the personal benefits of change can distinguish a successful change initiative from a frustrating failure.

So, while there are distinct differences in the leadership and interaction styles of physicians and non-physician executives, both face similar challenges, especially as change agents. Ultimately, successful healthcare leadership involves integrating clinical expertise and strategic and operational acumen to achieve optimal patient care and organizational performance.

45

Administrative Harm is Destroying the Practice of Medicine

"Rules and regulations, who needs them?
Throw them out the door."

— Graham Nash (lyrics), from "Chicago," sung by
Crosby, Stills, Nash & Young

Business entrepreneur and billionaire Michael B. Kim was quoted as saying: "Leadership without ethics is a body without a soul." Kim donated $25 million to his alma mater, Haverford College in suburban Philadelphia, Pennsylvania, to start a new Institute for Ethical Inquiry and Leadership. His goal is to renew society's focus on ethics, even dispatching "ethics missionaries" throughout the world.

A good first place to embed ethics missionaries is health care, where "administrative harm"—the negative impact on patients and health care providers caused by bureaucratic processes, policies, or inefficiencies within the health care system—is pervasive. Examples include unrealistic staffing models, burdensome regulations, out-of-touch administrators, lack of frank feedback to leaders, and unhelpful consultants. Administrative harm can manifest in excessive paperwork, rigid protocols that do not allow for individualized patient care, and resource limitations that prevent timely and adequate treatment.

Worse yet, there is no method of tracking these harms, mostly perpetrated by bottom-line-oriented hospital administrators. Given that there are approximately 10 administrators for every physician in the U.S., how *can* we effectively track these harms? Since the implementation of managed care in 1970, the number of doctors in the U.S. has increased by approximately 200 percent. In stark contrast, the number of health care administrators has surged by over 3,800 percent. During the same period (1970 to 2019), health care costs have escalated by 3,100 percent, rising from $353 per person in 1970 to $11,582 per person in 2019, adjusted for inflation.

Despite the significant expenditure on health care, the U.S. overall Global Health Security (GHS) index score in 2023 was 73.3 out of 100 points. This ranking is 69 out of 167 total countries rated and is even unfavorable compared to many third-world countries. The U.S. has the lowest life expectancy among large, wealthy countries while it far outspends its peers on health care. These poor rankings are partly a result of administrative harm, or what some also refer to as "management malpractice." As more funds are diverted to maintaining an inefficient administrative infrastructure, less money is available for actual health care services. This is a disgraceful situation.

The impact of administrative harm on patients can be seen virtually everywhere:

- Patients are missing out on successful disease management programs that have been subjected to budget cuts.
- Increasing patient transfers into hospitals with prolonged waits in emergency departments (ED).
- Increasing use of ED boarding of mental health patients, particularly those from racial and ethnic minority groups, leads to adverse outcomes, violence, and disparities in care.
- Lack of reliable data to determine when patients are medically ready for discharge.
- Lack of specialized staff or understaffing leads to unsafe practices and harm to patients (and staff).

- Insufficient patient information due to different electronic health record systems that don't communicate with each other.
- Duplicate records cause patients to repeat treatments and tests.
- Over-engineered systems are impacting patient flow.
- Delays in care are secondary to insufficient hospital and residential beds, lack of weekend services, and untimely responses to insurance authorization requests.
- Mergers that neglect local culture and lead to financial strain and hiring freezes.

Administrative harm can be considered a subtype of moral injury insofar as it often arises when health care providers feel they cannot provide the level of care they believe is necessary due to systemic constraints or administrative decisions. When practitioners are forced to navigate these administrative barriers, they may experience a conflict between their professional values and the realities imposed by the system. This conflict can lead to feelings of frustration, helplessness, and guilt, which are key features of moral injury.

Administrative harms are destroying the practice of medicine or at least taking away the pleasure and privilege of serving patients. In a 2011 editorial titled "The Quiet Epidemic," the authors focused on barriers to care imposed by insurers and pharmaceutical companies. They wrote: "The components of what we used to call comprehensive, multidisciplinary team care seem to have been replaced by only those services that are allowed or reimbursed. The world, at times, seems to have gone mad with senseless (at least from a clinical point of view) administrative rules."

The good news is that some harms may be preventable, largely through improved communication and collaboration between practitioners and administrators. The authors of a recent editorial wrote: "Administrators can listen to their clinicians and find ways to make it easier, not harder, for them to practice. They can also empower clinicians to identify problems that require solutions and speak up when interventions are not working. Given that U.S. medicine is less and less practiced in individual physician-run offices and more and more in larger practices and health systems in which physicians are employed, such efforts will be critical to avoid administrative decisions that cause more harm than benefit to clinicians and patients."

Another physician noted, "In an era when so many decisions are being made far away from patients, it's at the least ironic, but certainly unreasonable, that administrative decisions don't receive the same sort of scrutiny [as physicians]." Perhaps administrators should be rated on the morbidity and mortality of their own staff—those who remain at the end of the year and those who have been swept away for unethical decision-making and other reasons. Different turnover rates would be very telling. Unscrupulous decision-makers need not apply for the job of hospital administrator.

Who would have guessed that Michael Kim's first novel, *Offerings*, the story of an investment banker from Seoul who works on Wall Street and closely mirrors his own life, is now being made into a movie? His Institute for Ethical Inquiry and Leadership should be required training for all health care administrators. They should also adopt Kim's motto to live by: "Be grateful. Be humble. Be seated."

The Choice Between an "Episode" and a "Condition" is a False Dichotomy

How President Biden's disastrous debate
performance torpedoed his career.

Former House Speaker Nancy Pelosi said it is valid for people to ask whether Joe Biden's at-best poor, at-worst incoherent debate performance against Donald Trump on June 27, 2024, was just an "episode" or part of a "condition."

"I think it's a legitimate question to ask whether this is an episode or a condition," Pelosi said less than a week after the debate.

"It was a bad episode, no indication of anything serious," Biden told ABC News' George Stephanopoulos in an exclusive interview eight days after the debate. "I was tired. I didn't listen to my instincts in terms of preparation, and it was a bad night."

Biden has taken the bait that almost everyone else has taken, except those in the medical field who distinguish between an "episode" and a "condition." Critics have failed to adopt a perspective that acknowledges the complexity and variability of many medical conditions, which often present with both chronic and acute components.

A "condition" usually refers to an underlying health problem that persists over time. Examples include diabetes, hypertension, and chronic obstructive pulmonary disease (COPD). These conditions are characterized by their long-term nature and need for ongoing management.

An "episode," on the other hand, usually refers to a specific, usually temporary event or exacerbation of a condition. For example, a hyperglycemic crisis in a person with diabetes, a hypertensive emergency in a person with hypertension, or an acute exacerbation of COPD are all episodes. These episodes represent acute, often severe manifestations of the underlying chronic condition.

Let's give a few examples to explain this interaction:

1. **Asthma.** Asthma is a chronic respiratory condition characterized by inflammation and narrowing of the airways. People with asthma live with the condition for a long time, but they can experience acute attacks, known as asthma attacks or exacerbations. These attacks are periods when symptoms suddenly worsen and usually require immediate medical attention.

2. **Rheumatoid Arthritis (RA).** RA is a chronic autoimmune disorder that affects the joints. People with RA have ongoing joint inflammation and damage. However, they may also experience acute flare-ups, where symptoms such as pain, swelling, and stiffness intensify and require adjustments in treatment or more aggressive treatment.

3. **Heart failure.** Heart failure is a chronic condition in which the heart's ability to pump blood is impaired. Patients manage their condition with lifestyle changes and medications. However, they may experience acute episodes of decompensated heart failure, where symptoms such as shortness of breath, swelling, and fatigue suddenly worsen and often require hospitalization.

4. **Diabetes.** Diabetes is a chronic metabolic condition characterized by high blood sugar levels. While patients manage their blood sugar levels daily, they may experience acute attacks such as diabetic ketoacidosis (DKA) or hyperosmolar hyperglycemia state (HHS), which are serious and require immediate medical attention.

Mild cognitive impairment (MCI) fits well into the paradigm of chronic conditions with potential acute attacks. MCI represents a chronic neurological disorder characterized by a marked decline in cognitive abilities such as memory and thinking skills, but does not significantly impact daily life. This chronic nature means that individuals with MCI are at increased risk of developing more severe cognitive impairments such as Alzheimer's disease or other forms of dementia.

However, individuals with MCI may also experience acute attacks or exacerbations, often triggered by other factors. For example, an acute illness or infection, such as a urinary tract infection or pneumonia, may temporarily worsen cognitive function and lead to delirium or acute confusion. This condition is usually reversible with treatment of the underlying disease.

Medication effects may also play a role in acute cognitive impairment. Some medications, particularly those with anticholinergic properties or sedatives, can acutely impair cognitive function in individuals with MCI. Adjustment or discontinuation of these medications can sometimes reverse cognitive decline.

Psychosocial stressors, such as the loss of a loved one or major life changes, can temporarily worsen cognitive symptoms. Similarly, metabolic imbalances such as dehydration, electrolyte disturbances, or poorly controlled diabetes can lead to acute cognitive changes. Addressing these imbalances can often improve cognitive function.

Management of MCI includes strategies to slow the progression of cognitive decline and improve quality of life. This includes lifestyle interventions such as regular physical exercise, cognitive training, and a healthy diet, and medical management of cardiovascular risk factors such as hypertension, diabetes, and hyperlipidemia. Regular cognitive assessments are also important to monitor progression to more severe cognitive impairment.

Pressed by Stephanopoulos, Biden declined to take a cognitive exam, citing his schedule and workload as sufficient evidence that he could handle the job of president. He also cited his recent demanding international travel schedule and a "cold" as reasons for his debate crisis. I'm not saying Biden has MCI, but if it's true, it can be managed like flare-ups of other chronic diseases.

Preventing acute confusional episodes includes prompt treatment of infections and illnesses, regular review of medications to avoid medications that may affect cognitive function, and providing psychosocial support to manage stressors and provide a stable environment. Understanding and managing both the chronic aspects of MCI and potential acute episodes are important to providing comprehensive care for individuals with MCI. This approach is consistent with recognizing the interrelated nature of chronic conditions and their acute manifestations in medicine.

Chronic conditions often serve as the backdrop for acute attacks. Viewing them as separate entities oversimplifies the interconnectedness and dynamic nature of many medical conditions. It is well understood in clinical practice that patient care often requires a nuanced approach that considers both the chronic and acute aspects of a condition. Understanding this relationship is crucial to comprehensive care because it highlights the need for both long-term management strategies and acute intervention plans.

As we consider Biden's resignation from the 2024 presidential election, we can recognize the significant error he and his team made in allowing themselves to be confined to an "either/or" stance, essentially falling into a false dichotomy of being forced to decide between an "episode" and a "condition." While there are effective strategies for managing chronic conditions like MCI, there is no way to prevent a pathological liar from persisting in their deceit.

47

Navigating Patient Deception Requires Strategies for Enhancing Trust and Treatment Adherence

Deal with deceptive patients by gaining their trust and checking their compliance with therapy.

During my residency, I treated a patient with bipolar disorder. At the time (1981), the mainstay of treatment was lithium carbonate. Despite its potential side effects—such as thyroid and kidney issues, confusion, and others—it was, and continues to be, an effective mood stabilizer. One aspect I particularly appreciated was that serum lithium levels could be monitored reliably, with a therapeutic range for prophylaxis between 0.6–0.8 mmol/L and in acute treatment 0.8–1.2 mmol/L.

My patient's lithium levels were persistently low, but she insisted that she was taking the dose I had prescribed, which under normal circumstances should have yielded a therapeutic level. However, because my patient was doing well clinically, I decided to let it be. One day, I received a phone call from her daughter saying, "Mom is manic again." She was subsequently hospitalized, and it was then that I discovered my patient had been untruthful; she had been skipping most of her lithium doses. Naturally, I felt frustrated and deceived.

Any patient's deception is a challenging and sensitive issue that requires careful consideration and a balanced approach to the situation. A modicum of empathy and compassion is warranted even though your immediate reaction may be the opposite. Fostering an environment where patients feel safe to discuss their concerns and behaviors without fear of reprimand is crucial. Encouraging open dialogue can help patients feel more comfortable sharing their struggles with adherence. Ensuring that the patient fully understands the importance of medication adherence and the potential consequences of non-adherence is also essential.

Providing education about the disorder and the role of medication can empower patients to take an active role in their treatment. Continuing to monitor serum levels of medication when possible and other relevant parameters closely, along with regular check-ins, can help detect non-adherence early and provide opportunities to address it proactively. Patients with bipolar and other mental disorders may experience periods of impaired judgment or denial about their condition, which can influence their adherence to medication and their honesty about it.

Involving family members or caregivers in the treatment process can provide additional support for the patient. They can help monitor adherence and provide additional insights into the patient's behavior and well-being. My patients' daughter informed me that her mother liked the "high" that often accompanies mania, despite its possible destructive forces manifesting in risk-taking, sexual indiscretion, unwise investments, buying sprees and other sequelae.

I reflected on this experience as a learning opportunity important for professional growth. I considered how I might approach similar situations in the future and what strategies I could employ to improve patient adherence and communication. I realized that building a strong, trusting relationship with patients is crucial. I concluded that while deception can be disheartening, maintaining a non-judgmental and supportive attitude can help rebuild trust and improve future interactions. In fact, I continued to treat this patient well beyond my residency.

While her deception was understandably infuriating, it presented an opportunity to extend our relationship and actually enhance my approach to her treatment. It also marked the beginning of my interest in and understanding of the roots of deception and its myriad clinical presentations. Patients may have various reasons for not being truthful and deceiving healthcare providers, including fear of judgment, misunderstanding the treatment, or experiencing side effects they don't want to disclose. Understanding these behaviors can help practitioners to better diagnose and treat their patients.

One common way patients might deceive healthcare providers is by underreporting or overreporting symptoms. Some patients might minimize their symptoms to avoid the perceived stigma of certain conditions, out of fear of a serious diagnosis, or to avoid certain treatments or hospitalizations. Conversely, others might exaggerate or feign symptoms to obtain medications, avoid school or work, or secure disability benefits—so-called malingerers

Non-disclosure of information is another form of deception. Patients might withhold details about their medical history, including previous diagnoses, surgeries, or treatments, due to embarrassment or fear of judgment. They might also not disclose lifestyle choices such as smoking, alcohol consumption, drug use, or sexual behavior that could be relevant to their health. Additionally, as I learned, patients might not admit to not taking their prescribed medications or taking them incorrectly.

Falsifying information is also a concern. Patients might falsify self-monitoring data such as blood sugar readings, blood pressure logs, or weight to avoid lectures or additional interventions from their healthcare providers. Some might even invent symptoms or conditions to gain medical attention or sympathy.

Another deceptive behavior is doctor shopping. Patients might visit multiple healthcare providers to obtain additional prescriptions, particularly for controlled substances, without informing each provider of the others. They might also provide different histories to different providers to manipulate diagnoses or treatments.

Psychological factors can also lead to deception. Patients might be in denial about the severity of their condition and thus provide inaccurate information. Those with cognitive impairments might unintentionally provide inaccurate information due to memory or comprehension issues. Psychological factors are clearly at work in patients who intentionally report or fabricate symptoms in order to assume the patient role without obvious secondary gain—for example, patients with factitious disorders (Munchausen's syndrome).

Cultural and social factors can also play a role in patient deception. Some patients might withhold information due to cultural beliefs about illness, treatment, or the healthcare system. Social pressure can also lead patients to conform to norms or expectations, resulting in incomplete or inaccurate reporting.

Healthcare providers can take several steps to mitigate the impact of patient deception:

- **Build Trust**: Establishing a trusting relationship can encourage patients to be more honest.
- **Non-Judgmental Approach**: Using a non-judgmental and empathetic approach can help patients feel more comfortable sharing sensitive information.
- **Clear Communication**: Explaining the importance of accurate information for effective treatment can motivate patients to be more truthful.
- **Cross-Verification**: Using multiple sources of information, such as medical records, lab results, and input from family members, can help corroborate patient reports.
- **Routine Screening**: Regular screening for substance abuse, mental health issues, and other conditions can uncover discrepancies in patient reporting.

By being aware of the potential for deception and employing strategies to address it, practitioners can improve the accuracy of diagnoses and the effectiveness of treatments.

****

There is a denouement to this story. Many years later, after I had changed practice locations and transferred the patient to another psychiatrist, my phone rang.

"Dr. Lazarus," the caller asked?

"Yes," this is Dr. Lazarus, I replied.

"I found you!" the caller exclaimed.

It was my former patient, clearly experiencing a manic episode. Individuals with bipolar disorder sometimes go to great lengths to reconnect with past acquaintances and revive old friendships. After we exchanged a few pleasantries, I managed to persuade her to resume her lithium treatment and get in touch with her current psychiatrist. I'd like to believe she followed my advice due to our previous strong and trusting therapeutic relationship, although I cannot be entirely sure she complied.

48

Medical Gaslighting and Strategies to Combat It

Don't let the medical encounter turn into a one-sided affair.

The Gish gallop—named after American creationist Duane Gish, who challenged the science of evolution—is a rhetorical technique often used by a debater to throw out a fast string of lies, non-sequiturs, and specious arguments, so many that it is impossible to fact-check or rebut them in the amount of time it took to say them (think: Donald Trump). Trying to figure out how to respond makes the person look confused, because they don't know where to start grappling with the flood of lies that has just hit them.

It is a form of gaslighting.

The term "gaslight" originates from the 1938 play *Gas Light* written by British playwright Patrick Hamilton. The play was later adapted into a successful 1944 film titled "Gaslight," starring Ingrid Bergman and Charles Boyer.

In the story, a husband manipulates his wife into thinking she is going insane by gradually dimming the gaslights in their home and then denying that the lights are changing, among other deceptive tactics. This psychological manipulation leads the wife to doubt her own perceptions and sanity.

Gaslighting is real and widespread in medicine. According to the October 2022 SHE Media Medical Gaslighting survey, 72% of women experienced medical gaslighting. In addition to women, other vulnerable groups include people of color, members of the LGBTQ+ community, and older adults. Gaslighting makes patients seem or feel unstable, irrational, not credible. It makes them question themselves and their experience utilizing an imbalance of power between practitioner and patient.

Medicine is, unfortunately, full of that imbalance of power—in knowledge, time, and physicality. One is an all-knowing doctor (or advanced practice provider); the other is a lay person. The patient is in a gown; the doctor wears a white coat or is dressed business casual. There is a time imbalance in which patients live with their conditions sometimes for years yet healthcare workers must squeeze in a whole discussion of that condition in 10 or 15 minutes.

All of those imbalances are so powerful that they can even overcome a healthcare professional's knowledge and judgment when the healthcare professional is a patient. Many doctors and nurses who have experience heath care from the "other side" have written about being gaslit. Overwhelmed by the force of another healthcare professional, they come to doubt themselves and fail to trust in their own experience, which causes them to question themselves and their sanity. Just imagine how the experience of being gaslit feels for routine patients if it can feel that bad for people who work in the healthcare system.

Patients can be gaslit in various ways, such as dismissing or minimizing symptoms by attributing them to psychological causes without thorough investigation, contradicting a patient's account of their symptoms or medical history without evidence, or ignoring and belittling a patient's concerns or questions. These actions can deeply affect patients, leading to increased anxiety, depression, feelings of helplessness, and a significant erosion of trust in healthcare providers and the healthcare system as a whole. Moreover, it can result in delays in diagnosis and treatment, further compromising patient health outcomes.

Several factors apart from a power imbalance can contribute to the occurrence of gaslighting in medical practice. Implicit biases related to gender, race, age, or mental health can lead to dismissive attitudes towards certain groups of patients. Communication issues including poor interpersonal skills and a lack of empathy can also result in misunderstandings and dismissive behavior.

Addressing gaslighting requires increasing awareness among healthcare providers about the signs and impacts of their behavior. Correcting the underlying factors is crucial in preventing and mitigating gaslighting. This means training practitioners in empathy, active listening, and cultural competence, emphasizing a patient-centered approach that validates patient experiences and involves them in decision-making. Healthcare providers have an ethical duty to respect patient autonomy, provide truthful information, and avoid harm. Adherence to professional standards and guidelines that promote respectful and evidence-based patient interactions is essential.

Patients who feel as though they have been gaslit by healthcare providers can employ various strategies to advocate for themselves and ensure they receive appropriate care. One effective approach is to document everything meticulously. Keeping detailed records of medical interactions, including symptoms, dates, times, and specifics of conversations with healthcare providers, can provide a clear timeline and serve as evidence if needed.

Seeking a second opinion is another crucial strategy (refer to essay 13). Patients should feel empowered to consult another healthcare provider if their concerns are not being taken seriously. A fresh perspective can validate their experiences and provide new insights. Additionally, bringing a trusted friend or family member to appointments can offer emotional support and another perspective on the conversation. This person can help take notes and advocate on the patient's behalf.

Clear and assertive communication is essential. Patients should express their concerns and symptoms without minimizing them, using "I" statements to convey their feelings without sounding accusatory. Asking detailed questions about diagnoses, treatment options, and the reasoning behind medical decisions can help patients gain a better understanding and feel more involved in their care. Requesting written summaries of visits, including diagnoses, treatment plans, and follow-up steps, can also ensure clarity and provide a reference for future appointments.

Utilizing patient advocates or ombudsmen can assist in resolving concerns about care. These professionals can help navigate the healthcare system and mediate between patients and providers. Additionally, educating themselves about their symptoms and potential conditions can empower patients to ask more pointed questions and feel more confident in their interactions with healthcare providers.

If gaslighting persists, patients should consider reporting their concerns to the healthcare facility's administration or relevant regulatory bodies. Formal complaints can sometimes prompt necessary changes and accountability. Seeking emotional support from mental health professionals, such as therapists or counselors, can help patients process their experiences and build resilience. Patients who have been severely affected by gaslighting may require trauma-informed psychotherapy.

Connecting with others who have had similar experiences through support groups can provide validation, advice, and encouragement. These groups can be found online or through local community organizations. Finally, if a patient consistently feels gaslit by a particular provider, it may be beneficial to switch to a different practitioner or practice. Finding a provider who listens and respects their concerns is crucial for effective care.

In conclusion, gaslighting in medical practice is a serious issue that undermines patient trust and can lead to adverse health outcomes. By fostering a culture of empathy, respect, and patient-centered care, healthcare providers can reduce the risks of gaslighting and improve the overall patient experience. Patients should not persist with providers who engage in gaslighting; they should be equipped with strategies to counteract it.

Debaters are instructed to call out the Gish gallop by name, identifying their opponent and saying to the audience: "This is a strategy called the 'Gish Gallop'—do not be fooled by the flood of nonsense you have just heard." This declaration casts doubt on their opponent's debating ability for an audience unfamiliar with the technique, especially if no independent verification is involved, or if the audience has limited knowledge of the topics.

Taking affirmative action in one form or another is often the best way to deal with experiences that are consistently dismissed by the people who make you feel crazy.

49

The Synergy Between Clinical Pearls and Evidence-Based Medicine

Bridging practical wisdom and scientific rigor in medical practice.

The term "pearls of wisdom" in medicine refers to concise, insightful pieces of advice or knowledge that are valuable for clinical practice. These pearls often distill complex medical information into memorable, practical tips that can guide physicians and healthcare professionals in their day-to-day work. The origin of this phrase dates back to ancient times and is derived from the idea that pearls, being precious and rare, symbolize something of great value. In the context of wisdom, it implies that the knowledge shared is particularly insightful and worth remembering.

In medicine, "pearls of wisdom" are often passed down from experienced clinicians to trainees, much like how pearls are handed down through generations. These nuggets of information are typically succinct and easy to remember, making them effective teaching tools. They encapsulate essential clinical principles, diagnostic tips, treatment strategies, or patient management advice that can be quickly recalled in practice. For example, a common pearl might be, "When you hear hoofbeats, think horses, not zebras," which advises clinicians to consider common conditions before rare ones in their differential diagnosis.

The use of pearls of wisdom as a teaching tool is widespread in medical education. They are often shared during rounds, lectures, or informal discussions. These pearls help bridge the gap between theoretical knowledge and practical application. For instance, a senior physician might remind a junior doctor, "Always look at the patient, not just the monitor," emphasizing the importance of clinical assessment over sole reliance on technology. Another example could be, "Treat the patient, not the number," which cautions against focusing solely on laboratory results without considering the patient's overall clinical picture.

These pearls are valuable because they are born out of years of experience and are often learned through direct patient care. They can also serve to highlight common pitfalls and provide guidance on best practices. For instance, "If something doesn't fit, think about what you're missing," encourages clinicians to reconsider their diagnosis if the patient's presentation doesn't align with the expected clinical course.

Clinical pearls are part of the vast domain of experience-based medicine and seem to be most helpful in dealing with clinical problems for which scientific evidence and data from controlled clinical trials do not exist. However, just as the data in a clinical trial may lead to a drug's approval by the FDA with a "black-box" warning, the authors of a review article suggest that the pearl also come with a warning attached to it: "use of this pearl without analysis and without clinical judgment can be dangerous to your patients and to your intellectual development."

In other words, students (recipient of pearls) should accept pearls with caution and consider the observational data on which they are based. Likewise, teachers (givers of pearls) should follow guidelines for validity of their clinical pearls, including multiple observations and compatibility with existing data and practice location.

This advice leads to an interesting question: What is the relationship between clinical pearls of wisdom and evidence-based medicine (EBM)? The relationship is a nuanced one, to be sure, as both play crucial roles in modern practice but originate from different perspectives and approaches.

Whereas clinical pearls may not always be derived from rigorous scientific studies and can sometimes reflect anecdotal experiences or traditional practices, evidence-based medicine emphasizes the integration of the best available research evidence with clinical expertise and patient values. EBM involves systematic research, critical appraisal of the literature, and the application of findings to clinical practice. It aims to provide a more standardized and scientifically validated approach to patient care, reducing variability and improving outcomes.

The relationship between clinical pearls and EBM is complementary but can also be tension-filled at times. Clinical pearls often provide quick, actionable advice that can be used in the moment, while EBM requires a more methodical approach to integrating the latest research findings into practice. Ideally, clinical pearls should be informed by and consistent with the principles of EBM. For instance, a clinical pearl that advises "start low and go slow" with medication dosing in elderly patients aligns well with EBM principles, as it is supported by research on pharmacokinetics and the increased risk of adverse effects in this population.

To bridge the two, clinicians can critically evaluate the pearls they encounter, considering whether they are supported by the current scientific evidence. For example, a pearl like "Always rule out non-cardiac causes before diagnosing chest pain as a heart attack" should be evaluated in light of existing guidelines and research on chest pain management. When clinical pearls are consistent with EBM, they can serve as valuable reminders of best practices. Conversely, if a pearl contradicts current evidence, it may prompt a reevaluation of its validity and usefulness.

In practice, experienced clinicians often use a blend of both approaches. They rely on clinical pearls for quick decision-making and practical tips while grounding their overall practice in the principles of EBM. This hybrid approach ensures that patient care is both efficient and scientifically sound.

In summary, I'd like to leave you with a few pearls of my own:

- "Pearls of wisdom" in medicine are cherished pieces of advice that condense critical clinical insights into memorable and practical guidance.
- They serve as an effective teaching tool, enabling the transmission of essential knowledge and experience from seasoned clinicians to those still learning the ropes.
- Their enduring value lies in their ability to distill complex information into simple, actionable advice that can significantly impact patient care.
- Clinical pearls of wisdom and evidence-based medicine are interconnected yet distinct aspects of medical practice.
- Clinical pearls offer practical, experience-based insights that can enhance day-to-day decision-making, while EBM provides a rigorous, research-based foundation for clinical practice.
- When harmonized, they enable clinicians to deliver high-quality, patient-centered care that is both effective and grounded in the best available evidence.

Afterword

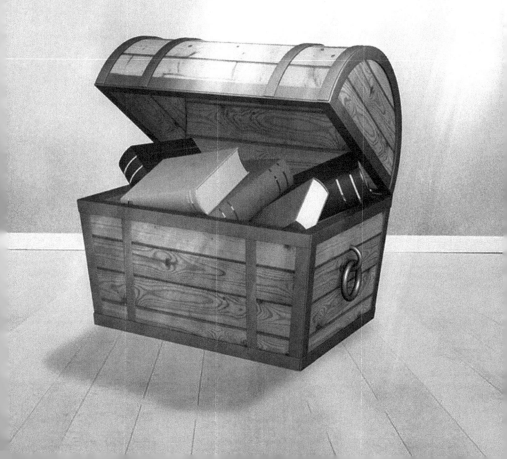

50

A Legacy of Action and Memories

It's all that you can't leave behind that matters in the end.

I mentioned in essay 37 that my wife and I recently downsized and moved into a house that's about half the size of our previous homes. This experience prompted me to reflect on the significant choices I made about what to leave behind while packing, and ultimately, what will remain after my passing.

For example, there is the legacy of my actions. The impact I have had on others through my personal and professional life will continue to resonate. My achievements, contributions, and the influence I've had on loved ones, patients, and colleagues will create a lasting legacy. Additionally, the ethical and moral principles I have upheld can inspire and guide others even after I am gone.

Also, the memories shared with loved ones will remain. The bonds I formed with family, friends, and colleagues are cherished and will be recounted by those who knew me. These personal relationships and shared experiences provide comfort and a sense of connection, allowing my presence to be felt long after my passing.

By considering these elements, I was able to capture the essence of what endures beyond a person's physical existence. I was able to definitively realize that upon your death, all that you can leave behind is the legacy of your actions and the memories shared with loved ones. Giving up personal possessions while downsizing, no matter how cherished those possessions were to me, became easier with the end goal in mind, i.e., working toward a legacy of actions and memories.

The Irish rock group U2 undoubtedly were contemplating the same issue when they released their 2000 masterpiece "All That You Can't Leave Behind." The album spawned hit singles like "Beautiful Day," "Stuck in a Moment You Can't Get Out Of," and "Elevation" which became the name of their subsequent tour. The album's title is taken from Bono's spoken word intro in "Walk On." He says, "The only baggage you can bring is all that you can't leave behind."

Emotional baggage traditionally refers to burdensome experiences and unresolved issues that hinder a person's ability to move forward in life. However, Bono's use of "baggage" refers to the foundational and integral parts of one's identity and life experiences that provide strength, wisdom, and resilience. These are the aspects that shape who we are in a positive way. This includes cherished memories, learned lessons, values, and relationships that enrich a person's life and contribute to their growth and resilience.

Bono's lyrics in "Walk On" encourage us to differentiate between the burdens that weigh us down and the essential elements that we carry with us for strength and guidance. The song addresses perseverance and reward and emphasizes the idea that in life, the most significant things we carry with us are the intangible, emotional, and meaningful aspects—our experiences, memories, values, relationships, and the essence of who we are. These are the things that define us and stay with us, regardless of our circumstances. Unlike material possessions or past traumas, regrets, and emotional scars that can create obstacles in forming healthy relationships and achieving personal growth, these are the true "baggage" that we bring along on our journey through life, as they are integral to our identity and cannot be easily discarded or stolen.

Several intangible and meaningful aspects of life are mentioned as the important "baggage" a person carries. The most important one is love: "Love is not the easy thing/The only baggage that you can bring." As the song progresses, Bono encourages the listener to get rid of excess baggage they have collected during their life's journey:

All that you fashion
All that you make
All that you build
All that you break
All that you measure
All that you steal
All this you feel
All this you can leave behind
All that you reason
All that you care (It's only time)
And I'll never fill up all my mind
All that you sense
All that you speak
All you dress up
And all that you scheme
All you create
All that you wreck
All that you hate

What we carry with us is particularly significant to me as a physician, especially as I near retirement. Throughout my career, I've tried to make a difference in my patients' lives through the care and compassion I provided and by leaving a strong clinical imprint on the pharmaceutical and health insurance industries. I hope my professional contributions, such as research, publications, and leadership in medical organizations will continue to benefit the field of medicine and future patients.

The mentorship and teaching I've offered to younger physicians, medical students, and other healthcare professionals have helped shape their careers and, by extension, the future of medical care. The relationships and bonds I've formed with colleagues, staff, and patients create lasting memories, carrying forward my influence and values. These elements represent the core values and experiences that define my professional life, and which cannot be taken away or left behind.

I would expect that most physicians my age can make similar comparisons, perhaps even those that extend beyond individual patient care to community health initiatives, public health advocacy, or medical outreach programs. The ethical standards and compassionate care they've practiced should set a benchmark for others in the field, influencing medical ethics and patient care standards.

As I transition into retirement, reflecting on these aspects can provide a sense of fulfillment and purpose. My career has left a significant mark on many lives. I can especially take pride in knowing that my actions, the memories shared with others, and especially my loving interactions with my family will continue to resonate long after I'm gone. I shall not leave any of it behind.

NOTES

Essay 1

1   *New York Times* article: https://www.nytimes.com/2022/08/31/opinion/ashley-judd-naomi-suicide.html
2   Werther effect: https://www.bmj.com/content/368/bmj.m575?ijkey=ef1ef161b1c66655f82261af0a01dbee92616034&keytype2=tf_ipsecsha

Essay 2

1   Lawsuits against the manufacturer of Gardasil: https://www.charlotteobserver.com/news/business/article286347750.html
2   Draft FDA guidance document: https://www.fda.gov/media/179593/download

Essay 3

1   John Coltrane's "A Love Supreme": https://www.friendsofjcmc.org/blog/2018/9/30/reflections-on-john-coltranes-a-love-supreme
2   Abraham Maslow's hierarchy of needs: https://www.simplypsychology.org/maslow.html

Essay 5

1   Chelsea Turgeon, MD quote: https://www.kevinmd.com/2024/02/how-medical-training-indoctrinates-toxic-beliefs-in-physicians.html
2   Ellen D. Feld, MD quote: https://jamanetwork.com/journals/jama/fullarticle/1817800
3   CEO quote: https://www.medscape.com/viewarticle/409812_4?form=fpf

Essay 6

1   Tod Stillson, MD "binary myth": https://www.kevinmd.com/2024/04/ dismantling-the-mythical-dichotomy-of-physician-career-options.html

Essay 7

1   Psychiatric maltreatment of patients: https://www.mattsmental healthmission.net/
2   Dr. "H. Anonymous": https://www.alphaomegaalpha.org/wp-content/ uploads/2021/03/2019-1-Lazarus.pdf
3   Vicarious trauma: https://www.aafp.org/pubs/afp/issues/2021/0501/ p570.html
4   Traumatic event exposure: https://www.ncbi.nlm.nih.gov/pmc/articles/ PMC4869975/
5   5. AA community centers: https://www.recoveryanswers.org/assets/Th e-Origins-of-Recovery-Community-Centers.pdf

Essay 8

1   Scholarly productivity and academic rank: https://shmpublications. onlinelibrary.wiley.com/doi/10.12788/jhm.3631

Essay 14

1   The origin of "publish or perish": https://garfield.library.upenn.edu/ commentaries/tsv10(12)p11y19960610.pdf
2   Gender inequality in academic medicine: https://jamanetwork.com/ journals/jamanetworkopen/fullarticle/2781617
3   Camille Paglia quote: https://www.jstor.org/stable/20163474?read- now=1#page_scan_tab_contents

Essay 15

1   Estimate of "alien earths": https://www.space.com/11188-alien-earth s-planets-sun-stars.html

Essay 16

1   Artificially intelligent scribes: https://catalyst.nejm.org/doi/full/10.1056/CAT.23.0404

Essay 17

1   Artificial intelligence used in breast mammography screening: https://pubs.rsna.org/doi/10.1148/radiol.232479

Essay 18

1   Neural mechanisms underlying emotional responses to music: https://www.researchgate.net/publication/23291396_Emotional_Responses_to_Music_The_Need_to_Consider_Underlying_Mechanisms

Essay 19

1   Statement from Done Global: https://www.donefirst.com/company/statement

2   Forbes Health quote: https://www.forbes.com/health/mind/best-online-therapy-for-adhd/

3   Senators' letter to Cerebral: https://www.klobuchar.senate.gov/public/_cache/files/2/e/2e36adce-7c6a-491f-87e6-a42262e16b65/CF3D6D0CF2D853FD17E1916DA2D95551.health-data-privacy-letter-to-cerebral.pdf

4   Prevalence of ADHD in adults: https://www.sciencedirect.com/science/article/pii/S0165178123003992?fr=RR-2&ref=pdf_download&rr=8178bea22f7642eb

5   Prevalence of depression in adults: https://jamanetwork.com/journals/jamapsychiatry/fullarticle/2671413

6   Prevalence of ADH in the psychiatric population: https://pubmed.ncbi.nlm.nih.gov/34061698/

7   Quote from Done's founder: https://www.linkedin.com/in/rujia/

Essay 20

1   Review article ("Physician Reluctance to Intervene in Addiction"): https://jamanetwork.com/journals/jamanetworkopen/fullarticle/2821497?utm_source=For_The_Media&utm_medium=referral&utm_campaign=ftm_links&utm_term=071724

Essay 21

1 Time to make a first impression: https://www.medcepts.com/first-impressions-33/

Essay 23

1 Memo from President Biden's physician: https://www.medcepts.com/first-impressions-33/
2 David Welky, PhD quote: https://www.washingtonpost.com/outlook/2020/10/13/roosevelt-lied-about-his-health-during-1944-election-with-stark-consequences/#click=https://t.co/TieEzqir6s

Essay 25

1 Near-death experience research: https://a.co/d/025Rg6b; and distressing experiences: https://med.virginia.edu/perceptual-studies/wp-content/uploads/sites/360/2017/01/NDE21_distressingfNDE-Psych.pdf

Essay 26

1 Spock's quote: http://www.chakoteya.net/StarTrek/22.htm

Essay 27

1 Quotes from "Space Seed": http://www.chakoteya.net/StarTrek/24.htm

Essay 28

1 NDP Analytics study: https://physiciansled.com/wp-content/uploads/2022/09/Economic-Impact-Report-2022-1.pdf
2 MD/MBA programs: https://jamanetwork.com/journals/jamanetworkopen/fullarticle/2806723
3 All physicians are leaders: https://www.physicianleaders.org/publications/books/all-physicians-are-leaders-reflections-on-inspiring-change-together-for-better-healthcare?v=31796288290887

Essay 31

1   Story shepherds of Northern Ireland: https://storyshepherds.org/asheville-wordfest-2022/

Essay 32

1   The Lancet Psychiatry article: https://www.thelancet.com/journals/lanpsy/article/PIIS2215-0366(15)00277-1/abstract
2   Prevalence of autism in a state psychiatric hospital: https://pubmed.ncbi.nlm.nih.gov/21846667/

Essay 33

1   Population distribution in the U.S. by generation: https://www.statista.com/statistics/296974/us-population-share-by-generation/
2   Zing Coach survey: https://www.zing.coach/fitness-library/healthy-or-not-attitudes-to-wellness-on-tiktok
3   Attention span of Gen Z students: https://www.keg.com/news/the-first-8-seconds-capturing-the-attention-of-gen-z-students; and compared to goldfish: https://time.com/3858309/attention-spans-goldfish/
4   Gen Z mental health: https://www.harmonyhit.com/state-of-gen-z-mental-health/; and openness about mental health: https://www.verywellmind.com/why-gen-z-is-more-open-to-talking-about-their-mental-health-5104730

Essay 36

1   reprinted with permission. *J Am Geriatr Soc.* 2024 (17 May);1-3. doi:10.1111/jgs.18976

Essay 38

1   The source of my instructor's quote: https://www.psychiatry.org/patients-families/hoarding-disorder/expert-q-and-a

Essay 39

1   Market estimate for self-help books: https://www.globenewswire.com/en/news-release/2023/11/30/2788922/0/en/Latest-Global-Self-Improvement-

Market-Size-Share-Worth-USD-81-6-Billion-by-2032-at-a-8-CAGR-C
ustom-Market-Insights-Analysis-Outlook-Leaders-Report-Trends-For
ecast-Segmentation-Grow.html

Essay 40

1 Medical Economic article: https://www.medicaleconomics.com/view/
6-reasons-why-doctors-get-scammed
2 Post by Victoria Strauss on Writer Beware®: https://writerbeware.
blog/2024/03/15/the-impersonation-list/
3 Financial fraud in the U.S.: https://bjs.ojp.gov/content/pub/pdf/ffus17_
sum.pdf

Essay 41

1 2016 World Series: https://www.cbssports.com/mlb/news/absurd-cub
s-indians-world-series-game-7-was-everything-we-love-about-baseball/

Essay 42

1 American Urological Association guidelines: https://www.auanet.org/
guidelines-and-quality/guidelines/testosterone-deficiency-guideline

Essay 44

1 MBTI profiles: https://www.jstor.org/stable/44950550

Essay 45

1 Michael B. Kim quote: https://www.haverford.edu/college-communications/
news/transformative-25-million-gift-michael-b-kim-85-establish-
haverford-s
2 Identifying and measuring administrative harm: https://jamanetwork.
com/journals/jamainternalmedicine/fullarticle/2820266
3 Ratio of administrators to doctors: https://pnhp.org/news/10-
administrators-for-every-1-doctor-we-deserve-a-better-healthcare-
system/
4 Health rankings of countries: https://www.statista.com/statistics/1376359/
health-and-health-system-ranking-of-countries-worldwide/

5   U.S. life expectancy: https://www.healthsystemtracker.org/chart-colle
    ction/u-s-life-expectancy-compare-countries/#Life%20expectancy%20
    at%20birth,%20in%20years,%201980-2022
6   "The Quiet Epidemic": https://jamanetwork.com/journals/jama/
    fullarticle/1104583
7   Editorial/quote about administrative harm: https://jamanetwork.com/
    journals/jamainternalmedicine/fullarticle/2820275
8   Physician quote about administrative harm: https://www.medpagetoday.
    com/special-reports/features/111028
9   Michael B. Kim's motto: https://www.inquirer.com/education/haverfor
    d-college-michael-kim-movie-board-chair-20240711.html

Essay 48

1   SHE Media survey: https://www.sheknows.com/health-and-wellness/
    videos/2687700/medical-gaslighting-statistics/#:~:text=Chloe's%20
    Most%20Recent%20Stories&text=According%20to%20the%20October%20
    2022,being%20blamed%20by%20your%20doctor.

Essay 49

1   Review article on clinical pearls: https://pubmed.ncbi.nlm.nih.gov/
    18821165/

ABOUT THE AUTHOR

Arthur L. Lazarus, MD, MBA, is a healthcare consultant, certified physician executive, and nationally recognized author, speaker, and champion of physician leadership and wellness. He has broad experience in clinical practice and the health insurance industry, having led programs at Cigna and Humana. At Humana, Lazarus was vice president and corporate medical director of behavioral health operations in Louisville, Kentucky, and subsequently a population health medical director in the state of Florida.

Lazarus has also held leadership positions in several pharmaceutical companies, including Pfizer and AstraZeneca, conducting clinical trials, and reviewing promotional material for medical accuracy and FDA compliance. He has published more than 400 articles and essays online and in scientific and professional journals and has written eight books, including four related to the field of narrative medicine.

Born in Philadelphia, Pennsylvania, Lazarus attended Boston University, where he graduated with a bachelor's degree in psychology with Distinction. He received his medical degree with Honors from Temple University School of Medicine, followed by a psychiatric residency at Temple University Hospital, where he was chief resident. After residency, Lazarus joined the faculty of Temple University School of Medicine, where he currently serves as adjunct professor of Psychiatry. He also holds non-faculty appointments as Executive-in-Residence at Temple University Fox School of Business and Management, where he received his MBA degree, and

Senior Fellow, Jefferson College of Population Health, Philadelphia, Pennsylvania.

Well known for his leadership and medical management skills, Lazarus is a sought-after presenter, mentor, teacher, and writer. He has shared his expertise and perspective at numerous local, national, and international meetings and seminars.

Lazarus is a past president of the American Association for Psychiatric Administration and Leadership, a former member of the board of directors of the American Association for Physician Leadership (AAPL), and a current member of the AAPL editorial review board. In 2010, the American Psychiatric Association honored Lazarus with the Administrative Psychiatry Award for his effectiveness as an administrator of major mental health programs and expanding the body of knowledge of management science in mental health services delivery systems.

Lazarus is among a select group of physicians in the United States who have been inducted into both the Alpha Omega Alpha medical honor society and the Beta Gamma Sigma honor society of collegiate schools of business.

Lazarus enjoys walking, biking, playing piano, and listening to music. He has been happily married to his wife, Cheryl, for over 40 years. They are the proud parents of four adult children and the grandparents of five young children.

Printed in the United States
by Baker & Taylor Publisher Services